T0146144

Narrative Psychiatry

Narrative Psychiatry

HOW STORIES CAN SHAPE CLINICAL PRACTICE

Bradley Lewis, M.D., Ph.D.
New York University
New York, New York

The Johns Hopkins University Press
Baltimore

"Mrs. Dutta Writes a Letter" © 1998 by Chitra Divakaruni

The Johns Hopkins University Press
2715 North Charles Street
Baltimore, Maryland 21218-4363
www.press.jhu.edu

Library of Congress Cataloging-in-Publication Data

Lewis, Bradley, 1956–
    Narrative psychiatry : how stories can shape clinical practice / Bradley Lewis.
        p. ; cm.
    Includes bibliographical references and index.
    ISBN-13: 978-0-8018-9902-7 (hardcover : alk. paper)
    ISBN-10: 0-8018-9902-8 (hardcover : alk. paper)
    1. Narrative therapy. I. Title.
    [DNLM: 1. Psychotherapy—methods. 2. Clinical Medicine—methods. 3. Mental
Disorders—therapy. 4. Narration. 5. Physician-Patient Relations. 6. Writing.
WM 420 L6763n 2011]
    RC489.S74L39 2011
    616.89'165—dc22

                                                                          2010023460

A catalog record for this book is available from the British Library.

*Special discounts are available for bulk purchases of this book. For more information,
please contact Special Sales at 410-516-6936 or specialsales@press.jhu.edu.*

The Johns Hopkins University Press uses environmentally friendly book materials,
including recycled text paper that is composed of at least 30 percent post-consumer waste,
whenever possible. All of our book papers are acid-free, and our jackets and covers are
printed on paper with recycled content.

CONTENTS

Preface   vii

1   *Listening to Chekhov*   1

2   *Narrative Medicine*   18

3   *Narrative Approaches to Psychotherapy*   32

4   *Narrative Psychiatry*   57

5   *Mrs. Dutta and the Literary Case*   75

6   *Mainstream Stories I:* BIOPSYCHIATRY, COGNITIVE BEHAVIORAL THERAPY, AND PSYCHOANALYSIS   86

7   *Mainstream Stories II:* INTERPERSONAL THERAPY, FAMILY THERAPY, AND HUMANISTIC THERAPY   104

8   *Alternative Stories:* SPIRITUAL THERAPY, EXPRESSIVE THERAPY, AND CULTURAL, POLITICAL, AND FEMINIST THERAPIES   121

9   *Doing Narrative Psychiatry*   144

10   *Critical Reflections*   157

Appendix: "Mrs. Dutta Writes a Letter," by Chitra Divakaruni   173
Notes   189
References   197
Index   211

PSYCHIATRISTS LISTEN TO STORIES more than anything else they do.[1] Their very first questions—"What brings you here?" and "What seems to be the problem?"—are open-ended invitations to a story. Patients respond to these invitations by telling psychiatrists about their life and their troubles. They give narratives of when their difficulties began, what they believe to have caused them, and what kinds of problem solving they have tried. Such stories may be rudimentary, they may be only partially worked out, and they may be confused and hard to understand. The patient may be perplexed enough to answer "I don't know why I came" or "I'm not really sure what's going on; my family sent me." Nonetheless, the patient's response to these initial questions always involves a story.

Follow-up questions aimed at particular symptoms also invite stories. Even the finely grained medical questions like "Do you have a history of diabetes?" or "Does depression run in your family?" involve stories. And the first clinical evaluation is only the beginning of the story-centric encounter between psychiatrist and patient. Later sessions and meetings deep into the treatment process, including those that involve only medication checks once every so often, are saturated with stories. "How have you been?" "What has happened since we last spoke?" "Are you having any side effects with this medication?" These questions all elicit stories from the patient.

Most psychiatrists have honed their extensive clinical experience with stories to the point that they are deeply skilled in the art of listening, and, for most psychiatrists, developing an ear for stories is a critical part of clinical expertise. In addition, there are formalized approaches to psychiatry that have specifically developed the role of stories for clinical care. Paul McHugh and Phillip Slavney, in particular, have spent decades nurturing a sophisticated approach to psychiatry that sees life stories as a fundamental tool of clinical work and clinical reasoning (McHugh and Slavney 1998).

Even with this dedicated interest in stories, psychiatrists have had little assistance in interpreting stories beyond their own clinical writings and clinical experience. Fortunately, the study of narrative outside psychiatry has grown exponentially in recent years, and it is now possible for psychiatry to gain considerable assistance in its capacity to appreciate stories and the role of stories for clinical work. Over the past thirty years, the study of narrative has been an important topic in a variety of fields, including literary theory, philosophy, history, cultural studies, religious studies, anthropology, and sociology. Furthermore, in the clinical worlds surrounding psychiatry, there is a growing movement in both medicine and psychotherapy to enrich and enhance clinical encounters through increased appreciation of narrative. This work has yielded fruitful and exciting work in the domains of narrative medicine and narrative psychotherapy.

In short, the turn to narrative is everywhere in the intellectual life surrounding psychiatry, and psychiatry has much to gain from this scholarly ferment. *Narrative Psychiatry* picks up this intellectual opportunity and develops the tools of narrative for psychiatry. I explore in detail the rise of narrative approaches to medicine and look closely at the ways narrative theory has been applied to psychotherapy. I also develop key philosophical and conceptual terms from literary theory to help psychiatrists achieve a deep appreciation of narrative for their work. Finally, I apply these terms to psychiatry, with specific attention to how narrative applies to the aspects of psychiatry that are similar to and different from medicine or psychotherapy.

This book is the product of my many years working and writing at the interface of clinical and theoretical work. I have also had the good fortune of teaching this material to students and residents at New York University for many years. Students and clinicians who take a narrative approach to psychiatry often find this material invaluable for understanding human life—particularly in the current moment of psychiatric history because narrative provides a much-needed counterbalance to contemporary efforts to ground psychiatry in genetics, bioscience, and neuropharmacology. Even though the biological turn in the psychiatry has brought a wealth of new perspectives and insights, it has also tended to leave psychiatric students and practitioners with limited conceptual tools for understanding empathic connections with people on a deep personal level. Knowledge about neurotransmitters and genetics does not help psychiatrists fully appreciate the interpretive dimensions of human problems—including the interpretive dimensions of neurotransmitters and genetics. To understand the complexities of human meaning, psychiatrists need additional resources.

At the same time, and just as important, narrative psychiatry also helps students and practitioners move beyond a binary logic that equates awareness of the limits of biopsychiatry with the legacy of antipsychiatry. This rigid either/or dichotomy paralyzes intellectual thought in psychiatry. It turns complicated theoretical and philosophical questions into shouting matches or pep rallies between two established teams: propsychiatry and antipsychiatry. This propsychiatry/antipsychiatry binary has worn out its usefulness, and narrative approaches are extremely helpful for moving beyond its limitations.

My interest in working through the possibilities of narrative psychiatry began after completing my previous book, *Moving beyond Prozac, DSM, and the New Psychiatry: The Birth of Postpsychiatry*. That book, which I think of as my "postpsychiatry book," explored the interface between psychiatry and postmodern philosophy. It joined a chorus of other philosophically oriented texts coming out at the same time that were concerned with psychiatry's rapid shift toward biology (Bracken and Thomas 2005; Brendel 2006; Double 2006; Fulford, Morris, Sadler, and Stanghellini 2003a; Ghaemi 2003; Radden 2004; Sadler 2004; Tamini and Cohen 2008). All of these books, in one way or another, were trying to understand how psychiatry has become so extensively preoccupied with biology and psychopharmacology at the expense of practically all else.

Making sense of psychiatry's sharp turn to biology has both personal and scholarly importance for me. The field's dramatic paradigm shift from psychoanalysis to biopsychiatry started in earnest in the early 1980s just after the American Psychiatric Association published the third edition of its *Diagnostic and Statistical Manual of Mental Disorders (DSM-III)*. These were the very years I was doing my psychiatric residency. Psychoanalysis, though on the decline, was still prominent, and the clash of the two paradigms created a training experience for me that Tanya Luhrmann perfectly captured in her book *Of Two Minds* (Luhrmann 2000).

Luhrmann, an anthropologist, undertook an ethnographic study of psychiatric training during the transition years and found that the two paradigms of biopsychiatry and psychoanalysis were not so much blending as existing side by side. The coexistence of the two paradigms created an educational environment for many psychiatric trainees, myself included, that would go back and forth between psychoanalytic worldviews and biopsychiatric worldviews depending on which mentor or seminar leader they happened to be seeing that day (or even that hour). Luhrmann argued that the two worldviews both had something to add, and she found that trainees got a fairly balanced exposure to both approaches. But the balance Luhrmann describes was short lived. Biopsychiatry was on the rise and psychoanalysis on the decline, and this trend has continued to the point where biopsychiatry is by far the most prevalent conceptual paradigm for psychiatrists today.

The standard explanation for the rapid emergence of biopsychiatry is simple: biopsychiatry represents scientific progress. Biopsychiatry, in this explanation, has triumphed over psychoanalysis because it comes closer to adopting methods of science and therefore is much closer to mirroring the truth of the real world. Psychoanalysis, in contrast, is little more than conjecture and hypothesis or, at worst, a dangerous collection of myths, superstition, and dogma. Either way, according to this standard logic, psychoanalysis had to fall in order to make room for the new truths of biopsychiatry.

This explanation never felt complete to me. I appreciated many of the insights from biopsychiatry, but I had also learned a great deal from my psychoanalytic mentors. As I looked more deeply into this paradox, my research for the postpsychiatry book brought me to a host of Continental philosophers and science studies scholars who questioned this standard explanation of scientific progress. Out of this group of thinkers, I found Michel Foucault's philosophy of science to be the most helpful. Foucault's theory of language and discursive practice is similar to Thomas Kuhn's theory of paradigms (Alcoff 2005, 211). Foucault, like Kuhn, was keenly interested in how prevailing paradigms of thought shift through time. For Foucault, real-world discoveries play a part in the formation of new paradigms—not anything can be said, and Foucault is not an "anything goes" relativist—but the real world is far too complex and multidimensional for this to be the only explanation. Yes, the real world accommodates and resists different possible ways of understanding it, and, yes, different knowledge formations yield different real-world capacities. But the real world alone does not determine knowledge. The real world does not come with tags on it or with predetermined frames and models with which to approach it. Humans must make these choices.

Thus, to understand new knowledge formations, one must also consider the social context of knowledge construction. Foucault took this insight and went on in his later work to add an articulation of *power* to help understand these social forces. For Foucault, the power dynamics at play during a paradigm shift (or what Foucault would call a discursive shift) are a major determinant of how the new conceptual system will form. To understand why a discursive shift happens, one must understand not only its material capacities but also the power dynamics surrounding the shift.

Applying Foucault's perspective to the paradigm switch in psychiatry from psychoanalysis to biopsychiatry suggested that, although biopsychiatry has its truths, so too does psychoanalysis. The truths and capabilities of biopsychiatry and those of psychoanalysis may not be the same, but neither can be entirely dismissed as myth or superstition. Each approach has learned something important about human psychic life. From a postpsychiatry perspective, the shift from psychoanalysis to biopsychiatry represented not so much "progress" as a shifting power balance that favored the emergence of biopsychiatry. In this shifting power balance to biopsychiatry, new material capacities emerged, but at the same time some of the wisdom of psychoanalysis was watered down or lost.

There are many ways to understand the shifting power dynamics in favor of biopsychiatry, and there are many changing social forces that one could point to—including the pharmaceutical industry, National Institute of Mental Health funding for neuroscience, managed care, competition with other provider groups, and so on. In the postpsychiatry book, I argued for the development of a cultural studies of psychiatry genre to help sort through these many issues (Lewis 2006b, 80–97). And contemporary scholarship from the humanities and social science is doing just that. Recent examples of the cultural studies of psychiatry genre include literature and disability studies scholar Lennard Davis's *Obsession: A History,* psychologist and cultural historian Gary Greenberg's *Manufacturing Depression: The History of a Modern Disease,* literature scholar Christopher

Lane's *Shyness: How Normal Behavior Became a Sickness*, anthropologist Emily Martin's *Biopolar Expeditions; Mania and Depression in American Culture*, communication studies scholar Majai Nadeson's *Constructing Autism: Unraveling the "Truth" and Understanding the Social*, and sociologist Jackie Orr's *Panic Diaries: A Genealogy of Panic Disorders* (Davis 2007; Greenberg 2010, Lane 2007; Martin 2007; Nadeson 2005; Orr 2006). This list only scratches the surface, and it seems clear that cultural studies of psychiatry are on a rapid growth curve. We can expect many more works from this genre in the near future.[2]

As informative as I have found cultural studies of psychiatry genre to be, I have also found it to be of limited use in the clinical setting. The cultural studies genre can tell you a great deal about the larger frames of psychiatry but not much about how individual people make personal choices to navigate and negotiate these larger cultural frames. After I finished the postpsychiatry book, the most frequent questions I received from clinical readers were: "What do you do differently in your clinical work with these insights from postpsychiatry?" and "How does postpsychiatric work change your clinical practice?" I had no particularly good answers for these questions. They are too finely grained for the broad "paradigms and power" perspectives of postpsychiatry. Just because you can point to power dynamics at play in the emergence of the available paradigms does not tell you which paradigm to choose. For Foucault, all knowledge is infused with power, so knowledge/power awareness does not in itself disqualify knowledge. Knowing the particular power dynamics can be part of how one assesses a paradigm, but it does not in itself determine the value of the paradigm for a particular person at a particular time.

Thinking through these more finely grained clinical questions, I found that narrative theory provided the optimal bridge between postpsychiatric cultural studies and clinical practice. Compared with postmodern theory and cultural studies, narrative theory focuses much more detailed attention on individual stories and individual lives. Narrative theory offers a rich language for understanding how linguistic frames and metaphorical structures get incorporated into lived experience and personal identity. Narrative theory helps connect the dots between large paradigms, like biopsychiatry or psychoanalysis, and the intimate details of personal life stories. It helps us see how people use and in some ways are used by available paradigms to make sense of their lives and the lives of others.

But narrative theory is not an easy domain to use for clinical work because narrative theory exists in so many varied contexts and contains so many complex threads and components. Foucault's work and the larger postmodern cannon are of little help for understanding narrative theory, and for that reason I shifted philosophical ground for this project. To anchor this project, I've moved from Foucault's work on discursive structures to Paul Ricoeur's work on narrative theory. Ricoeur is an ideal philosopher to anchor work in narrative psychiatry because his meticulous and painstakingly referenced corpus moves from his early work in phenomenology, through his own discursive and poststructuralist turn, to his final work on narrative theory and human identity. The longevity of Ricoeur's efforts allowed him to come through the other side of phenomenology and postmodern theory to think through in impressive detail the vicissitudes of what he calls "narrative identity."

Without Ricoeur's richly synthetic efforts, an interdisciplinary medical humanities book like this that applies narrative theory to psychiatry would be not be possible. I would forever need to work out philosophical details without being able to make applications to psychiatry. But, by standing on the shoulders of Ricoeur's work and mixing in a Foucauldian twist, the task of application is much more feasible. That said, however, this book is not a secondary text on Ricoeur, nor does it constantly tack back to his work alone. As in my previous book, I continue to take advantage of a host of literary and philosophical scholarship relevant to this topic. For readers who are philosophically minded (in particular for philosophy and psychiatry readers), I encourage them to engage in Ricoeur's work directly for fruitful extension and development of the many theoretical and philosophical arguments at play in this work.

In my first chapter, "Listening to Chekhov," I begin the process of developing a narrative frame for psychiatry through a close reading of *Ivanov*, a play by Anton Chekhov. I start this project with Chekhov because he brings together in one author the combined wisdom of a writer, a physician, and a person who has depression. His play gives us a subtle and sophisticated presentation of human sadness without the need to close down the interpretation to a single interpretive frame. Chekhov's approach is a kind of narrative psychiatry before the letter. Much of the task of today's narrative psychiatry will be to catch up to the wisdom of Chekhov.

Chapters 2 and 3 explore recent historical trends toward narrative in psychiatry's two closest neighboring disciplines: medicine and psychotherapy. These two sister disciplines are so close to psychiatry that we might usefully think of psychiatry as part medicine and part psychotherapy. Indeed, one of the quickest ways of understanding psychiatry is to say that it is coidentified with both medicine and psychotherapy. Psychiatry's swings between the two sister disciplines come from how it is identified in some ways with hard-nosed medical types and in other ways with tender-minded therapists and counselors. This leaves psychiatrists sometimes performing like medical physicians, sometimes like psychotherapists, sometimes combining the two. Interestingly, for our work here, cutting-edge work over the past few decades in both medicine and psychotherapy has taken a "narrative turn." These chapters consider this trend by asking three main questions: What is it about the history of medicine and psychotherapy that has made the turn toward narrative so compelling? How might psychiatry learn from an appreciation of these narrative developments in closely related clinical domains? And which parts of narrative theory have been most useful for these domains? It is in the last of these questions where I rely most heavily on Ricoeur's philosophy.

Chapter 4 brings the insights from the first three chapters together to consider the emergence of narrative psychiatry. Until recently, psychiatry has been left out of the narrative turn in medicine and psychotherapy for a variety of reasons, the most important of which is psychiatry's efforts over the same period of time to be as scientific as possible. This effort has tended to cut psychiatry off from important humanistic trends in both medicine and psychotherapy. The tides are clearly changing, however, and the time is ripe for psychiatry to take its own turn toward narrative. This chapter explores how psychiatry got to its current state and how the narrative turn provides an invaluable tool for contemporary psychiatrists. It also differentiates narrative psychiatry from either narrative medicine or narrative approaches to psychotherapy. Although there are similarities in these fields, there are important differences to be understood as well.

Chapter 5 shifts focus from theory to application to review the advantages of using literary fiction as a pedagogic tool for psychiatry. It begins a discussion of a case example drawn from a short story by Chitra Divakaruni, "Mrs. Dutta Writes a Letter." A copy of the story is included as an appendix, and during the course of this chapter I ask readers to pause to read this lovely story. If students of narrative psychiatry can see the role of narrative for making sense of a particular case history, they have a much deeper appreciation of narrative work. Divakaruni's story, like many literary fiction stories, provides an excellent source for what I call "literary case histories." Divakaruni gives us a rich contextual background for her characters—much richer than most clinical narratives. The very richness of this background shows how possible it is to tell many different kinds of stories about Mrs. Dutta's situation. As with Chekhov's approach to Ivanov, we consider these many possibilities over the rest of the book without insisting on a single truth.

Mrs. Dutta's "case history" therefore serves as a backdrop in the next three chapters for a discussion and application of an array of mainstream and alternative clinical stories that emerge in the many different models of psychiatry. The approaches I consider in Chapter 6 are mainstream options of biopsychiatry, cognitive behavioral therapy, and psychoanalysis. In Chapter 7, I consider the less common mainstream options of interpersonal therapy, family therapy, and humanistic therapy. In Chapter 8, I consider the more alternative options of spiritual therapy, expressive therapy, and cultural, political, and feminist therapies.

All of these clinical and alternative stories may be seen as larger cultural narratives through which clinicians help patients reauthor their stories in more helpful ways. Clinical tales like these do not stay in the clinics; they permeate culture, and they are permeated by culture. Paying close attention to the models of psychiatry through the lens of narrative theory provides a wealth of resources for understanding human problems and difficulties. To make this point clearer, in these chapters I consider how the different approaches to psychic problems might be relevant for Mrs. Dutta. Looking at Mrs. Dutta's situation through different clinical models reveals a vast array of life options she might choose from. Narrative psychiatrists need to be familiar with these options because the more stories they know, the more use they can be in the process of helping people restory their lives.

Chapter 9, "Doing Narrative Psychiatry," considers how a narrative psychiatrist might help Mrs. Dutta navigate the many options before her. In addition, this chapter connects the dots between narrative psychiatry and recent work in bioethics and the recovery movement in psychiatry. I argue that a narrative approach to psychiatry is deeply synergistic with bioethics and recovery in its spirit and goals. Indeed, only through joining colleagues in medicine and psychotherapy in a "narrative turn" can psychiatry coherently practice ethical and recovery-oriented clinical work.

In the final chapter, "Critical Reflections," I consider the many objections people have to narrative psychiatry. The ideas of narrative psychiatry are often counterintuitive and can leave people with a host of critical concerns. By working through these objections, we gain more ease with the language of narrative and more familiarity with how psychiatrists can take a narrative turn without falling into the many pitfalls that people might imagine. Once psychiatrists become comfortable with the narrative turn, they will have an expanded and rejuvenated set of tools for helping people understand the stories of their lives and make changes for the better. In the end, helping people make informed choices about the options for storying and restorying their lives is at the heart of psychiatric practice. Narrative tools are invaluable for this goal.

A modified version of chapter 1 was published in *Literature and Medicine* under the title "Listening to Chekhov: Narrative Approaches to Depression." Copyright © 2006 Johns Hopkins University Press. This article first appeared in *Literature and Medicine* 25.1 (2006): 46-71. Reprinted with permission by The Johns Hopkins University Press. A modified version of chapter 2 was published in the *Journal of Medical Humanities* under the title "Narrative Medicine and Healthcare Reform." Used with kind permission from Springer Science+Business Media (Online First, 5 November 2010; www.springerlink.com/content/104920/?Content+Status=Accepted). An earlier version of chapter 4 appeared in Kaplan and Saddock's *Comprehensive Textbook of Psychiatry*, 9th edition.

Narrative Psychiatry

CHAPTER ONE

Listening to Chekhov

D ESPITE THE SERIOUSNESS of what we call mental illness in contemporary times—both its pervasive incidence and the extensive suffering it causes—this is an era that struggles with how to understand the
multiple interpretations of psychic suffering and psychic difference. Most
psychiatric discourse embraces a biological model that articulates mental
illness as a medical disease involving neurological pathology. This model
uses disease logics, like the commonly held notion of a "neurochemical
imbalance," and the expected solution lies in pharmaceutical interventions.[1]
The number of prescriptions written using this perspective is phenomenal.
One example is Prozac: between 1987 and 2002 (the year Prozac came off
patent), the number of new prescriptions for the drug exceeded 27 million. When that number is combined with prescriptions for the multiple
"me too" drugs Prozac inspired—the class of antidepressants known
as selective serotonin reuptake inhibitors (SSRIs)—the total reaches 67.5
million in the United States alone.[2] These numbers suggest that almost
one in four people in the United States was started on a Prozac-type drug
between 1987 and 2002.

Simultaneous with this dramatic epidemic of prescriptions, there has
been ardent criticism of all this brain focus in psychiatry. Many critics
argue that the biological interpretation of mental difference is wrong
because it is either too reductionistic or too simple (or both). Scholars repeatedly denounce the reductionist approach of biopsychiatry for deny-
ing the complexity of human life. We are more than our bodies and brains,
they argue; we are also our experiences, our hopes, our dreams, our histories, our cultures, our politics. Versions of this argumentative style show
up in popular critiques of biopsychiatry, such as *Toxic Psychiatry*; *They
Say You Are Crazy*; *Madness, Heresy, and the Rumor of Angels: The Revolt against the Mental Health System*; and *Blaming the Brain*.[3]

Philosophical psychiatrist Edwin Wallace sounds a similar note when he criticizes psychiatry's diagnostic manual. Wallace, like almost everyone who seriously evaluates the manual, faults it for its oversimplified "claim to atheoreticism" (Wallace 1994, 81). He argues that psychiatry's relentless pursuit of atheoretical simplification flies in the face of the twentieth century's "most respected philosophers of science," who have all held that idealized theoretical neutrality is a logical and empirical impossibility. As Wallace points out, it is not merely scientific assumptions and theories that we can't escape but also "social, political, and moral philosophical ones as well" (1994, 81). Any attempt to avoid these complications does "violence to large arcs of the person and ignores or derides theoretical purviews and therapeutic modalities that can be necessary or lifesaving" (1994, 85).

Certainly, there is value in these critiques as a first step in moving beyond an idealization of biopsychiatry. It is important to highlight that biopsychiatric simplifications reduce complex reality to whatever fits into a simple scheme. We should also remember that reductions "forget" about the complex, which means that the complex is often surprising and disturbing when it inevitably reappears later on. However, it is equally important to be suspicious of denunciations of reduction and simplicity because these critiques can become too sterile, too easy, too disturbingly agreeable and self-satisfying. It can become a morally too comfortable place to be, and it leaves a great deal to discover. As science studies scholars John Law and Annemarie Mol put it, "We need other ways of relating to complexity, other ways for complexity to be accepted, produced, or performed" (Law and Mol 2002, 6).

It is time to move beyond probiopsychiatry interpretive models and also beyond antibiopsychiatry critiques of reductionism and simplicity. We cannot idealize the dominant biological discourse as the only way to think about mental difference, nor can we do no more than accuse biological interpretations of being too reductionistic. We need a new approach to psychiatry that can hold in tension the value of biological models (even when they are reductionistic and oversimplified) while at the same time putting these models into a greater perspective. What we need, as I argue throughout this book, is a narrative approach to psychiatry.

Turning to Chekhov

Developing a narrative frame for psychiatry requires us to step back from contemporary biopsychiatry and its critics, and there is no better place to begin than with the work of Anton Chekhov. Chekhov gives us the combined wisdom of a writer, a physician, and someone who suffered his own mental anguish. Moreover, Chekhov did most of his work just before the emergence of psychiatry as a modern medical discipline, which means that his perspective was not hardened in advance by well-established disciplinary traditions and their critiques.

As a writer, Chekhov was a deep and rare genius of the ordinary and the everyday. His stories and plays, often of sadness and woe, gave European literature a subtle and richly ambiguous world of psychological, moral, and social contemplation. Because Chekhov was also a physician, he approached these tales not only with the eye of a literary master but also with the experiences of his medical science training and his life of clinical encounters. Chekhov was, in other words, as devoted to medicine as he was consumed by literature. Shortly after medical school, he traveled more than eight hundred kilometers across Siberia to study the harsh medical conditions of an infamous penal colony. When he returned, he set up and maintained a general medical practice, kept meticulous records, and at one time was appointed district public health officer during a raging cholera epidemic. Chekhov acknowledges in an autobiographical statement that he persistently used his medical training in his creative work: "My knowledge of natural sciences and scientific methods has made me careful and I have always tried, when possible, to take into consideration the scientific data [when I write]" (Coulehan 2002, xiii).[4]

In addition to his extraordinary skills in literature and medicine, biographers suspect that Chekhov had his own periods of depression: despair, loss of confidence, and loss of pleasure in his life. His worst suffering came just after his brother, Kolia, died of tuberculosis when Chekhov was a young man, but the echoes and permutations of sadness run throughout Chekhov's life. Much of his suffering may have revolved around his premonitions of death. Like his brother, Chekhov died young from tuberculosis (at the age of forty-four). His first bout of hemoptysis occurred in 1884, the year he graduated from medical school. After that, episodes of coughing up blood recurred regularly each year. Although Chekhov did not speak publicly of his disease until near his death, he must have known fairly early on that he was dying from consumption. In all likelihood, both the sadness and the wisdom that pervade Chekov's work are connected to his awareness of death and these early intimations of mortality.[5]

As one might suspect with this background, Chekhov's writings contain many portrayals of psychic distress. The short story "The Fit" features a law student who relapses into depression after witnessing the exploitation and cruelty of brothel life. The play *Uncle Vanya* portrays the chronic despair of its protagonist, Vanya. In "A Doctor's Visit," a young girl falls into a state of anxiety, weeping, and sobbing related to the desolation of her surroundings. "Ward Number 6" tells the story of a medical superintendent's decline and eventual admission into his own psychiatric asylum. And in "The Black Monk," Chekhov depicts the strange hallucinations and despair of Kovrin, a young philosophy student who is fatally ill with tuberculosis.[6]

But Chekhov's most concentrated study of mental distress and difference comes from his early play *Ivanov*, in which the lead character, Nikolai Ivanov, suffers from a deep and profound sadness. The play reads much like a psychiatric case study. Dr. Chekhov presents Ivanov's difficulties with the reflective empathy of a master clinician and the subtlety of a great writer. He does not romanticize Ivanov's troubles (indeed far from it), nor does he force his interpretation into a single pathological frame. Chekhov presents Ivanov with all the simplicity and complexity that realistic fiction requires. This approach to "the case" of Ivanov is exemplary in the study of psychiatry because, all too often, psychiatric case studies come to us in a predetermined explanatory frame. Chekhov resists this temptation, and as a result, his case study of Ivanov is an extremely useful guide for us today.

Ivanov's situation can be summarized as follows: he is a thirty-five-year-old married Russian landowner who has been in excellent health all his life. But over the past two years, he has gradually sunk into increasing sorrow and despair. He struggles with unshakable feelings of melancholy and even suicidal preoccupations that are so severe that, by the play's end, he takes his own life.

The question that runs throughout Chekhov's play is perhaps the most obvious one: How should the events leading up to Ivanov's death by self-inflicted gunshot wound be interpreted? What, in short, is wrong with

Ivanov? Although the question may be straightforward, the subtleties of Chekhov's answers are anything but, and these subtleties are particularly difficult for contemporary audiences to apprehend. Thanks to the tremendous influence of today's medical models of mental suffering, modern audiences are likely to interpret Ivanov as biologically/neurologically depressed.

Consider what happened when psychiatrist Peter Kramer, the author of the 1990s best seller *Listening to Prozac*, went to a production of the play at the Lincoln Center. From his *New York Times* review it is clear that, even though Kramer is one of the more subtle of today's biologically oriented psychiatrists, when he listens to Ivanov's troubles he hears a straightforward case of clinical, or medical model, depression (Kramer 1997). Kramer finds Ivanov to be a veritable catalog of diagnostic signs and symptoms. Ivanov is persistently sad, irritable, and bored with life. He has marked feelings of guilt and worthlessness, inability to sleep, lack of appetite, and lack of sexual desire for his wife. In addition, Ivanov is severely suicidal. For Kramer, Ivanov has all the key symptoms that, according to the American Psychiatric Association's *Diagnostic and Statistical Manual of Mental Disorders*, 4th edition (*DSM-IV*), indicate a "Major Depressive Disorder, Single Episode, Severe, without Psychotic Features—diagnostic code 296.23" (American Psychiatric Association 1995, 347).

Not only does Kramer see Ivanov as biologically depressed, but also he makes the claim that his own clinical ear, his way of listening to Ivanov, has become the current cultural dominant.[7] For the "contemporary ear," Kramer argues, the play has been "sapped of any moral consequence" (Kramer 1997). Persistent sadness is a chemical imbalance, and "suicide is part of the disease. . . . Suicide is what the death certificate says when one dies of depression" (1997). End of analysis. To diagnose Ivanov's depression, Kramer seems to feel there is no need for further interpretation—except perhaps to seek out Ivanov's genetic flaws and biological predispositions. There is no need to ask, "What is Ivanov so depressed about?" or "What does Ivanov's suffering mean in a larger frame?" For Kramer, whatever the reasons for Ivanov's sadness, they are insufficient to account for his clinical depression. As the title of his review makes clear, what Ivanov needs today is an antidepressant.[8]

But Kramer's confident biological interpretation—useful as it may be in some circumstances—misses exactly what is most interesting about *Ivanov*.

Kramer gives no personal or historical context and disregards entirely the fact that *Ivanov* is set in a time of great political upheaval and social malaise in Russia: the generation before the 1917 revolution, a period Chekhov biographer Donald Rayfield calls "one of the richest and most contradictory periods in Russia's political and cultural history" (Rayfield 1997, xvi). And, even more important, Kramer ignores how the play centers not so much on Ivanov himself but on the whole question of interpreting and categorizing humans. As drama critic Richard Gilman asserts, the central point of the play "isn't Ivanov's behavior in itself but the range of reactions to it and, by extension, the whole question of how much we can know about ourselves and other people" (Gilman 1995, 67).

What is most fascinating about *Ivanov* is that almost every character has an opinion about Ivanov's problems, and throughout the play they offer diverse, wildly incommensurable interpretations of Ivanov. As Chekhov states in a letter to his brother, the play's originality comes not from its subject matter but from his own refusal to take an authorial position on the meaning of the play: "I have not introduced a single villain or a single angel (though I have not been able to abstain from fools): nor have I accused or vindicated anyone" (quoted from Hare 1997, vii).[9]

Thus, another understanding of Chekhov's play is that it is not about medical depression at all but, rather, the indeterminacy of interpretation. On this reading, *Ivanov* takes its place alongside Dostoevsky's work as an example of what Mikhail Bakhtin calls polyphonic fiction. For Bakhtin, the many voices and simultaneous points of view contained within Dostoevsky's fiction create a "polyphonic world" that destroys "the established forms of the . . . *monologic* (homophonic) European novel" (Bakhtin 1994, 90).[10] In a similar vein, Chekhov's polyphonic portrayal of Ivanov does not present an omniscient point of view, nor does it privilege any particular character's interpretation of Ivanov. Chekhov structures the play to highlight the multiplicity of meaning and the possibility of respecting the interpretive diversity of the characters. Looking more closely at the play's many perspectives on Ivanov, we get a clearer sense of what this might mean.

First, there is Borkin, the estate steward, who interprets Ivanov not as constitutionally depressed but as a "whining neurotic" (Chekhov 1967, 1.2.32).[11] Borkin believes Ivanov should drop all his melancholy talk, grow up, and start making some money. After all, Borkin exclaims to Ivanov, "you're not a schoolboy" anymore (3.8.29). In contrast, another character, Zinaida, Ivanov's best friend's wife, formulates Ivanov's sadness in a very different way: "Can you wonder darling? [Sighs] The poor man made a ghastly mistake—marrying that wretched Jewess and thinking her parents would cough up a whacking great dowry. It didn't come off. When she changed her religion they cut her off and cursed her, not a penny did he get. He's sorry now it's too late" (2.3.29–33). For Zinaida, Ivanov's sadness is the result of profound regret and lost expectation. From her perspective, Ivanov ruthlessly manipulated his wife for a dowry he never received, and he organized his life around that cold calculation. As a result, his regret is his just reward: his moral payback for treating his wife so callously.

Sasha, a young woman in the village, is in love with Ivanov and also sees his plight very differently. Sasha understands the problem to be not that Ivanov is callous and manipulative but that he is too kind and generous for his own good: "Ivanov's only fault is being weak and not having enough go in him to chuck out . . . Borkin. . . . He's been robbed and fleeced left, right and center—anyone who liked has made a packet out of Ivanov's idealistic plans" (2.3.78–82). Furthermore, Sasha sees Ivanov as lonely and forlorn. He has fallen out of love with his wife, through no fault of his own, but he hasn't the heart to break off the marriage. Sasha even has a treatment recommendation. "I understand you," she tells Ivanov. "You're unhappy because you're lonely. You need someone near you that you love and who'll appreciate you. Only love can make a new man of you" (2.4.14–16).

Anna, Ivanov's wife, agrees with none of these interpretations. Instead, she has a cathartic theory of Ivanov's troubles. For Anna, the problem is that Ivanov has failed to properly grieve for his many life disappointments. In other words, Ivanov needs to go through the work of mourning and come through to another side. This process, which psychoanalyst George Pollock calls "mourning-liberation," would allow Ivanov to heal through a proverbial welling up with tears (Pollock 1989). As Anna puts it, Ivanov should spend time alone with her in the dark clarity of night: "You can tell me all about how depressed you are. Your eyes are so full of suffering. I'll look into them and cry, and we'll both feel better" (1.4.55–57).

But Lyebedev, Ivanov's best friend, sees things very differently. Lyebedev puts Ivanov's despair in a social-historical context: "I don't know, old man. It did look to me as though your various troubles had got you down, but then I know you are not one to—it's not like you to knuckle under. . . . You know what? It's your environment that has got you down" (3.5.88–90, 97–98). Lyebedev believes that Ivanov's sadness comes from his social surroundings, which represent and are symptomatic of a broader cultural malaise, or what contemporary philosopher Susan Bordo calls a "crystal-lization of culture" (Bordo 1993, 139). Bordo uses this phrase to go be-yond the most liberal of clinical biopsychosocial formulations. The issue is not simply that psychiatric conditions have cultural expression and a social context. They do, of course. But, for Bordo, psychopathologies must be not only be culturally contextualized but also understood as symptom-atic articulations of deep cultural tensions and power imbalances. Psycho-pathologies, far from being anomalies or aberrations, are "characteristic expressions" of the cultural fault lines in which they develop (1993, 139). They signal and crystallize much of what is wrong with the culture of their formation.

While Ivanov the character quickly rejects an environmental inter-pretation, *Ivanov* the play does not. Throughout, as in most of Chekov's plays, there is a detailed description of the wane of the landed class, the rise of the business class, and the stale paralysis and anomie with which the gentry respond to it all. Indeed, in *Ivanov* it is not just Ivanov who is affected; many of the characters complain of boredom, lack of energy, and loss of pleasure. At a party, for example, we hear characters say, "Lord I'm bored stiff" (2.1.42), or "Don't you ever get tired of sitting around like this? The very air's stiff with boredom" (2.3.88–89). One guest even ex-claims, "This is all such a crashing bore, I feel like a running dive into a brick wall. God, what people!" (2.9.5–6). The air of depression and gloom found in so many of the men in the community provokes Sasha to exclaim, "There's something wrong with you all, and no mistake. The sight of you's enough to kill the flies or start the lamps smoking. Yes, there's something wrong—I've told you thousands of times and I'll go on telling you—something wrong with you all, wrong, wrong, wrong!" (2.3.103–7).[12]

But what does Ivanov have to say about his sadness? It turns out that even he feels conflicted about how to understand the depression he has. Sometimes Ivanov reduces his troubles to laziness and weakness of the will: "Laziness is laziness," he tells Sasha; "weakness is weakness—I can't find any other name for them" (4.8.68). In a soliloquy, he continues in this vein by calling himself a "nasty, miserable nobody" (3.4.1). But in talking to his friend Lyebedev, he works out an alternate, and detailed, formulation of what in contemporary U.S. culture we might call "burnout" or "midlife crisis." Ivanov explains that he was full of energy and enthusiasm in his youth: "I believed in different things from other people, married a different sort of wife, got excited, took risks . . . and was happier and unhappier than anyone else in the country" (3.5.98–100). All that activity has overstrained him. As he explains, "Those things were my sacks, I heaved a load on my back and it cracked. At twenty we're all heroes, tackle anything . . . but by thirty we're tired and useless" (3.5.100–103).

But Ivanov is inconsistent with this explanation as well. At a later point in the play he tells Lyebedev, "I won't try to explain myself—whether I'm decent or rotten, sane or mad. You wouldn't understand" (4.10.1–3). In this interpretation, Ivanov's perspective resembles Kramer's medical model, and he presents himself as having something like a medical disease: "I'm quite ill," he tells Yevgeni Lvov (the young village doctor). "I'm irritable, bad-tempered and rude. . . . I've headaches for days on end, I can't sleep, and my ears buzz. . . . I'm so mixed up, I feel paralyzed, half dead or something. . . . I don't know myself what's going on inside me" (1.3.55–56, 72, 88). At one point, he even says, "My brain doesn't obey me, nor my arms or legs," and he falls into weeping (3.4.13–14). Here, Ivanov sees his sadness as having no meaning, as being outside any human integrative frame—except of course the interpretive frame of bodies, brains, and medical science. From this biological model, Ivanov's depression comes out of the blue and exists at the status of pathophysiology, much like a heart attack or an idiopathic seizure.

Despite all the ambiguity within the play, there is one character, Dr. Lvov, who stands apart in his adamant certainty of his opinion about Ivanov's melancholia. It is with this character that Chekhov portrays, with full force, his negative authorial judgment: Lvov is the "the fool" Chekhov could not resist including. Lvov imagines himself to be an earnest, high-minded, dedicated physician with an intense social conscience. But the play's other characters do not see him, or his profession, in the same light. As one character says, "Doctors are like lawyers, only lawyers just rob you, while doctors rob you and murder you too" (1.3.1–3). Lvov comes across to many of the characters as priggish and self-righteous. "Oh, he's virtue incarnate," someone says mockingly of him, "can't ask for a glass of water or light a cigarette without displaying his remarkable integrity" (2.4.85–88).

Lvov's perspective on Ivanov turns out to be the harshest and most pathological of the play. Lvov finds Ivanov's melancholia and his related disinterest in his wife detestable. He labels Ivanov "insensitive, selfish, cold . . . heartless" (1.5.22) and an "unmitigated swine" (4.10.40–41). Lvov tells Ivanov that Anna "who loves you is dying . . . she hasn't long to live, while you—you are so callous . . . I do most thoroughly dislike you" (1.5.23–27). Lvov's scorn is at first met by Ivanov with weary admissions of blame and appreciation for Lvov's seemingly neutral concern. Within the context of the play, however, Lvov's neutrality is much less clear. There is constant tension regarding whether Lvov is in love with Anna and whether his interpretations of Ivanov are merely self-serving attempts to win Anna's affections.

Whatever Lvov's motivations, the more he presses his perspective, the more Ivanov loses patience with him. In one of the climactic scenes of the play, Ivanov exclaims to Lvov in exasperation: "Think a little, my clever friend. You think I'm an open book, don't you? I married Anna for her fortune, I didn't get it, and having slipped up then, I'm now getting rid of her so I can marry someone else and get *her* money. Right? How simple and straightforward. Man's such a simple, uncomplicated mechanism. No, doctor, we all have too many wheels, screws and valves to judge each other on first impressions or on one or two pointers. I don't understand you, you don't understand me and we don't understand ourselves. A man can be a very good doctor without having any idea what people are really like. So don't be too cocksure" (3.6.72–81). Ivanov scolds Dr. Lvov primarily because he oversells his diagnosis. Dr. Lvov fails to have humility in his perspective. He insists that he knows the truth of Ivanov's situation, and he behaves as if a human being is fully understandable—like a pulley or a mouse trap. And this is also the reason that Dr. Lvov becomes "the fool" in the play.

As harsh as this critique of Lvov may sound, Ivanov's advice to him is relevant for aspects of today's psychiatry, particularly the tremendous hype and promotion surrounding contemporary medical models of psychic difference and distress. But it is important to be clear exactly what is being critiqued here. Both in the play and in the extension of the play to today's psychiatry, the issue is not the medical interpretation in and of itself but the overconfidence with which it is asserted. Chekhov makes clear that the problem with Lvov's interpretation is not that it is wrong in any simple way, which is why Ivanov does not actually dispute the content of Lvov's claims. What Ivanov critiques is his dogmatic and cocksure certainty. As far as Lvov's specific interpretation goes, like everyone else in the play, he picks out elements of Ivanov's story and arranges them together into a plausible whole. That is not the problem. Likewise, it is not the problem for contemporary medical model interpretations like Kramer's. The play also contains data that support medical model perspectives on Ivanov's troubles. The problem is not either of these perspectives and the possible insights they might bring but the dogmatism and the hype with which they are held. The problem is the cocksure self-confidence of Lvov and Kramer's attitude.[13]

Such hype and overconfidence are blind to the possibility of multiple interpretations because they narrow meaning down to a single option. Dr. Chekhov counters Dr. Lvov's certainty with the challenge of a polyphonic world and with the multiplicities of consciousness and experience. Dr. Chekhov challenges Dr. Lvov to appreciate the possibilities of interpretative diversity. In this way, Dr. Chekhov's message is equally imperative for today's biopsychiatry. If biopsychiatry listened more closely to *Ivanov* the play, instead of narrowly reading Ivanov the character, it would throw its *DSM*-led interpretations (and its drive for antidepressant "cures") into the ring with a myriad of other interpretations. It would not foreclose other, equally vital understandings of melancholia and suffering.[14]

Developing a Narrative Frame for Psychiatry

With Chekhov's work in mind, we can recognize the need for an approach to mental illness that includes our current biological model (albeit in a more humble form) but also significantly refines this model. Single-minded biological models of depression are not enough. But what alternate model is Chekhov using that allows him to appreciate, rather than try to close down, interpretive diversity? Chekhov does not tell us. *Ivanov* is not an expository treatise on mental illness or a theory of mental illness; it is an imaginatively created case history. Chekhov leaves it up to the reader to put this case study into an interpretive frame.

Chekhov's model can best be understood as a narrative one. By this I mean that Chekhov is aware that there is no "one truth" of Ivanov's life and that there can be many plausible narrative interpretations of Ivanov's troubles. Chekhov also understands that which narrative interpretations (or which combination of interpretations) one selects matters immensely. For example, Borkin's interpretation that Ivanov needs to grow up and quit whining suggests that Ivanov should approach the world through Borkin's business values and priorities. Sasha's narrative reading of the lack of love in Ivanov's life implies that a new marriage will help him recover from his sadness. And so on with each different interpretation. These different interpretations are not simply ideas or random meaning structures. They are guides for action, and actions have consequences. A narrative frame that sets up a world with multiple truths hardly means that all truths are relative. Which truth we choose matters deeply.

Chekhov's narrative frame for depression likely emerged from his personal experience of combining medicine and literature. Chekhov famously describes the relationship between his two occupations in this way: "Medicine is my lawful wedded wife, and literature my mistress. When one gets on my nerves, I spend the night with the other. This may be somewhat disorganized, but then again it's not as boring, and anyway, neither one loses anything by my duplicity" (Chekhov 2004, 107). Chekhov uses this unfortunately sexist imagery to evoke his lived experience of moving back and forth between the two positions of medicine and writing. Through this constant movement, Chekhov broke out of the standard frame of most medical thinking to develop a narrative frame.

Chekhov's dual positions of doctor and writer produced diametrically opposed relationships to the role of narrative in representation. In his occupation as a doctor, Chekhov's task was to background narrative frame and to view his patients from a positivist model of objectivity. But this positivist stance (which continues to subtend most of medicine and psychiatry today) was not Chekhov's only position. As a writer, he worked from an opposite position that foregrounds narrative frame. In other words, he inhabited a practice that highlights the impossibility of telling a story without a point of view.

Contemporary physician-writer Abraham Verghese articulates this dual position in his discussion "The Physician as Storyteller." Speaking to fellow physicians at the American College of Physicians, Verghese explains that, "as physicians, most of us become involved in the stories of our patient's lives . . . we become players in these stories. Our actions change the narrative trajectory . . . and our patient's stories come to depend heavily on repetition of what we say" (Verghese 2001, 1012). Verghese argues that the inescapable thesis for medicine is threefold: "1.) *story* helps us link and make sense of events in our lives; 2.) we as physicians *create* stories as often as we record them . . . ; and 3.) we are characters in [these] various stories, walking on and off the stage in tales that take place in our hospitals and clinics" (2001, 1012; Verghese's italics).

Verghese points to examples by which physicians can reach this level of narrative awareness through years of attentive practice, but he argues that the more direct route is through combining the practice of medicine with the narrative tools that the writer possesses, or what Verghese calls the "storytelling craft" (2001, 1013). He explains that during his own initial immersion in the writing process he read closely and widely about the craft of writing. He found that the pillars of writing invariably involved the author's selection and organization of *metaphor, plot*, and *character*. For Verghese, making these selections is "fundamental to good writing in the same way that internal medicine skills rest on understanding the mechanisms behind dyspnea, edema, polyuria and other cardinal manifestations of disease" (2001, 1014).

Chekhov's combination of the storytelling craft and medical practice seems to have brought him to a similar narrative frame. When Chekhov includes physicians in his plays and short stories, they are hardly the voice of transparent objectivity. They represent one voice among many, one story among an array of stories. They may well be important to the plot, but they are hardly the positivistic truth.[15] As Verghese puts it, physicians are "storytellers, storymakers, and players in the greatest drama of all: the story of our patients' lives as well as our own" (2001, 1016).

Kathryn Montgomery Hunter, in her book *Doctors' Stories: The Narrative Structure of Medical Knowledge*, echoes this same sentiment: "Narrative of any length and fullness or speculative force inevitably pulls against medicine's commitment to objective scientific study of human illness" (Hunter 1991, 166). In making the case for a narrative understanding of medicine, Hunter explains that what is needed is a means of moving away from the illusion "of objectivist, scientific reportage" and toward an acknowledgment that medical case histories are "humanly constructed" accounts: "Two things are essential: first, both tellers and listeners must recognize the narrator of the case history as contextually conditioned, and, second, the lived experience of the patient must be experienced" (1991, 166).

Narrative emphasis on the contextually conditioned nature of knowledge, even medical knowledge, inevitably creates some ambiguity of interpretation. Though some might find this ambiguity troubling, Chekhov seems to revel in it.[16] Indeed, literary critic Karl Kramer refers to the frequent interpretive uncertainty in Chekhov's work as his "stories of ambiguity" (Kramer 1979, 338). Kramer's reading of Chekhov finds unresolved paradox structured into many of his stories. Through a study of subsequent drafts of Chekhov's work, Kramer argues that Chekhov often deliberately reworks a story so that it cannot be read through a simple monologic lens. The ambiguity comes from the way Chekhov sets up contradictory readings from parallel passages throughout a given story. The result is a story that can be interpreted in several different ways. Although one interpretation may appear more plausible than another, which often happens, no single reading will adequately account for the whole fabric of these stories. As Kramer puts it, that in and of itself "is sufficient to establish [Chekhov's stories of] ambiguity" (1979, 338).

This reading of Chekhov's writing fits perfectly with *Ivanov*. Throughout the play, as we saw earlier, each of the characters offers different narrations of Ivanov's sadness. From a perspective of multiple and ambiguous interpretations, the question to ask is not simply, which story is true? But, instead, what are the consequences of each story? And what kind of life will follow from inhabiting these stories? Even if there is no essential or singular essence to Ivanov's sadness, Ivanov arguably needs a story for his sadness. He can crystallize a provisional subjectivity around his sadness only through inhabiting a story and, to borrow a phrase from Freud, "working through" the implications of that story.[17]

From Antireductionism to Narrative Multiplicity

Peter Kramer is certainly right in his reading of *Ivanov* that today's era of biological psychiatry has cosmopolitan culture charging headlong into increasing brain science and brain interventions. But even as this happens, it is hard to escape the persistent feeling that we, as a culture, are missing something important. It is hard to escape the nagging suspicion that if we primarily study our brains, and primarily intervene by altering our neurotransmitters, we will become increasingly naive about the multiple meanings of psychic life at the same time that we are increasingly victim to psychic troubles. Yet even though it is time to move beyond biological models, we cannot embrace the dominant critical discourse of antibiopsychiatry that simply accuses biological models of being "too reductionistic." Instead, we need an approach that recognizes the value of reductionistic interpretive frames, including biopsychiatry, while avoiding the trap of simultaneously idealizing them. Narrative psychiatry, along with its core theory of narrative multiplicity, provides just that approach.

What I am arguing here is that we move from an antireductionst critique of biopsychiatry to a narrative multiplicity critique. But what would that mean? The difference between Kramer's celebration of biopsychiatry, the standard antireductionistics critique of biopsychiatry, and Chekhov's narrative approach to psychiatry is that Chekhov values complexity without denigrating simplicity. In *Ivanov*, Chekhov respects rather than denounces the characters' oversimplifications of Ivanov. Chekhov resists, in other words, a normative view of simplicity. He helps us see a world where alternative (and inevitably simple) interpretations are not so much wrong or bad but different. Chekhov does not denigrate the characters' reduction of Ivanov's sadness into simple formulas. Each character presents seemingly viable interpretive options. Lvov comes under the most criticism, but, as I mentioned earlier, this comes from his dogmatism, not from the potential viability of his interpretations.

How can we scaffold a position that recognizes the limitations of simplicity without simultaneously giving normative preference to complexity? How can we articulate the value of both simplicity and complexity? We can begin by recognizing that simple reductions become less problematic when we multiply them. Moving from a single order to multiple orders, from a necessary order to a variety of orders, undermines the dichotomy between simple and complex. By adopting a narrative frame the trope of violence gives way to the trope of narrative multiplicity. Multiplicities of metaphors, characters, and styles—not to mention multiplicities of models, perspectives, paradigms, and discourses—hold in tension both the values of simplicity and those of complexity. Narrative interpretive multiplicity recognizes that each simplicity necessarily fails to capture complexity. Each simplicity selects and organizes highly idiosyncratic cuts from the data. Each simplicity, in other words, is necessarily limited. These limited, unavoidably simplistic perspectives, however, are less of a problem when they multiply. When simplicity multiplies, instead of becoming hegemonic, it becomes one of many. Through multiplication, each simplicity loses the violence of totalitarian control.[18]

Conclusion

When we apply narrative interpretive multiplicity to psychiatry and mental illness, new forms of wisdom and flexibility emerge. Narrative multiplicity hardly embraces an "anything goes" relativity, but it does create a conceptual structure where ontological questions (e.g., What are the core features of psychic life?) and epistemological questions (e.g., What is the best method to study people?) are not fixed in advance. Different answers may emerge, depending on related ethical questions (e.g., What kind of people do we want to be? and What kind of life worlds do we want to create?). Different understandings of the core features of people and different methods of inquiry about people yield very different kinds of people and very different kinds of life experiences. There are multiple ways to interpret human life. Making judgments between these different ways largely depends on the consequences and desired values. In short, there are multiple paths to wisdom and a meaningful life.

When we adopt Chekhov's narrative approach to psychic suffering and difference, we move beyond biopsychiatry and its reductionist critiques, and we recognize that simplification and reduction—even when they take the narrative frame of biopsychiatry—are not the problem. The problem is the temptation of dogmatism and the refusal to appreciate an array of narrative simplifications. Accordingly, the goal of narrative psychiatry is not to denigrate single interpretive solutions for their simplicity, nor is it to take single solutions and make them complex. The goal is to increase our appreciation of alternative solutions, be they simple or complex. The goal is openness to a range of options and to the richness and variety of psychiatric experience.[19]

By sidestepping a deeply problematic probiopsychiatry/antibiopsychiatry binary, narrative psychiatry allows for a subtle appreciation of the many truths of psychiatry without overvaluing any of these truths as absolute. The next step after appreciating this philosophical point is to work out in more detail what it means for clinical life and clinical encounters. Fortunately, although the concept of narrative is relatively new in psychiatry, narrative approaches have become increasingly prevalent in both medicine and psychotherapy. Psychiatry can get a tremendous leg up on the meaning of narrative for clinical life by taking a close look at the recent narrative turns in both of these closely related domains.

CHAPTER TWO

Narrative Medicine

M ANY IN PSYCHIATRY may fear that a turn to narrative will risk alienating their hard-nosed medical cousins. They may think to themselves, "With the recent decade of the brain, the growth in 'hard' science research, and the explosion of pharmacological interventions, we are finally starting to get some respect from our medical colleagues. We are no longer a 'soft' specialty, one that is not 'really medicine.' We can hold our heads high, wear white coats, and monitor blood pressures and body mass index without seeming silly. If we take a narrative turn, won't we once again be seen by our medical colleagues as a pseudodiscipline—out of touch with the tough-minded realities of the brain and science?"

As anxiety provoking as that thought may be for psychiatrists, there is a good chance that a narrative turn for psychiatry would have just the opposite effect, that it would increase psychiatry's reputation rather than diminish it. Why? Because psychiatry's wholehearted embrace of neuroscience and pharmaceutical treatments has become a single-minded obsession that can make psychiatry look absurd, even a little mad, in the eyes of many of its peers. And, more important, the leading edge of medicine has already taken a narrative turn. Yes, we are in a paradoxical moment when medicine is more open than psychiatry to the human and the storied aspects of clinical work. As counterintuitive as it may seem, by taking the narrative turn, psychiatry does not risk "getting away" from medicine as much as it gains the possibility of "catching up" to medicine.[1]

A Brief History of Medicine

To understand the recent narrative turn in medicine, I shall tell a story that puts it in context and helps us understand the felt need for narrative work in today's medical practice. This story (like all stories) could be told with many beginnings, middles, and ends. The way I tell it starts not with Hippocrates or the many medical luminaries to follow him (such as Galen and Osler) but with Abraham Flexner—a former schoolmaster with no background in medicine. It goes something like this.

In 1908 the Carnegie Foundation for the Advancement of Teaching chose Flexner to head up a commission to assess U.S. medical education. At the time, most American medical schools were two-year "proprietary" schools owned by local doctors and unaffiliated with universities. Teaching varied enormously, and the scientific standards were not a high priority. Flexner was picked to report on these medical schools on the strength of his connections; his brother was director of the Rockefeller Institute for Medical Research—an institution with much to gain from the commission's eventual findings (Hiatt 1999). Flexner began his investigation by setting a benchmark for medical education based on the then current practices in Germany and the few U.S. schools that followed these practices. The German approach placed priority on university education and scientific research, which for Flexner was the cutting edge of medical progress. Using this model as a guide, Flexner eventually concluded that U.S. medical training needed a wholesale overhaul.

In the process of his report, Flexner narrowly defined the proper goals of medicine as the "attempt to fight the battle against disease" (Flexner 1910, 23). He argued that the future of pathology, therapeutics, and medicine depends on those trained in the methods of natural science. Clinicians must, in short, be "impregnated with the fundamental truths of biology" (1910, 25). As Flexner reasoned, "The human body belongs to the animal world. It is put together of tissues and organs, in their structure, origin, and development not essentially unlike what the biologist is otherwise familiar." Humans, like animals, are "liable to attack by hostile physical and biological agencies; now struck by a weapon, again ravaged by parasites" (1910, 25).

Flexner's analogy between humans and animals meant to him that the biological sciences provided the core content for all medical education. Consequently, he argued for medical student admission requirements, what we now call "pre-med," that concentrated on chemistry, biology, and physics. Flexner's first-year curriculum for medical school itself included anatomy, histology, embryology, physiology, and biochemistry, and the second year consisted of pharmacology, pathology, bacteriology, and physical diagnosis. Flexner's third and fourth years took the student to the hospital setting for clinical experience in the use of the stethoscope, palpitation, and percussion along with laboratory and microscopic skills in the study of excretions, secretions, and tissues.

Flexner's 1910 report was so successful that it transformed U.S. medical schools and created the basic structure for medical education today. Despite this institutional success, however, over time increasing numbers of physicians and scholars gradually realized that Flexner's approach to medicine—with its near-exclusive interest in the body, biology, and natural science—had a fundamental flaw. Humans are not the same as animals. In addition to having bodies, organs, and tissues, they live meaning-centered lives and have complicated emotional and historical relations with their bodies. Flexner's vision of medical education created physicians richly sophisticated in the animal part of medicine, biological variables, and biological interventions but who all too often lost touch with the human aspects of health care and the clinical encounter (Odegaard 1986).

By the 1970s and 1980s, meaningful resistance to Flexner's exclusive preoccupation with biology began to emerge. George Engel argued for an expanded "biopsychosocial" approach to medicine, which included not only the patients' bodies but also their psychic life and their social context (Engel 1977, 1980). Eric Cassell redefined the proper goals of medicine not as the battle against disease but as the tending to human suffering (Cassell 1982). And Ian McWhinney urged medicine to adopt a "person-centered" approach, which "should aim to understand the meaning of illness for the patient as well as provide a clinical diagnosis" (McWhinney 1986, 873).

In addition to these new clinical models of medicine, medical scholars took increasing interest in the role that humanities and interpretive human sciences could play in health care. Medical scholars began opening their knowledge base to inquiry coming from philosophy, anthropology, and literature. Several journals in these new interdisciplinary areas rapidly appeared: *Hastings Center Report* (1975), *Journal of Medical Ethics* (1975), *Man and Medicine* (1975), *Ethics in Science and Medicine* (1976), *Journal of Medicine and Philosophy* (1976), *Culture, Medicine, and Psychiatry* (1976), *Theoretical Medicine* (1981), *Literature and Medicine* (1981), *Social Science and Medicine* (1983), and *Journal of Medical Humanities* (1989).

Much of the early work from philosophy and medicine focused on ethical quandaries of the clinical encounter, particularly the dilemmas of conflicting values between physician beneficence, patient autonomy, and social justice. High-profile cases, like the Karen Ann Quinlan case, dealing with high-drama issues like the right to die captured the imagination of many. But more fundamental to the daily life of physicians, philosophers of medicine also argued that medical practice itself, in its everyday encounters with patients, must be understood not primarily as biological science. It must be understood first and foremost *as a moral relationship*. Internist and medical philosopher Edmund Pellegrino put it this way: "Medicine is a special moral enterprise because it is grounded in a special personal relationship—between one who is ill and another who professes to heal" (Pellegrino 1982, 156).

Medical philosophers turned to a branch of philosophy known as phenomenology to better understand the meaning of illness and the moral core of healing. The founder of phenomenology, German philosopher Edmund Husserl (1859–1938), who did much of his work around the same time as Flexner's report, called for a reorientation of European science toward human meaning and subjective life. For Husserl, the core flaw in Europe's Enlightenment science heritage was its obsessive pursuit of the objective while simultaneously neglecting and denigrating the subjective. The insistent exhortation of European science to "be objective" (familiar to all students of today's science-dominated medicine) led to an ignorance of human subjective experience and created a way of life out of touch with human needs, goals, desires, suffering, and meaning. Writing on the eve of the Nazi atrocities, Husserl argued that one-sided European objectivism had become so dominant that it had caused a crisis not only in science but also in Western humanity. For Husserl, "the 'crisis of European existence,' talked about so much today and documented in innumerable symptoms of the breakdown of life, is not an obscure fate, an impenetrable destiny; rather it becomes understandable and transparent against the background of the teleology of European *history* that can be discovered philosophically" (Husserl 1970, 299).

The only solution for the crisis of objectivism was a radical return to the phenomena of experience. Husserl's phenomenology begins by setting aside taken-for-granted presuppositions about the world to study lived experience: what is given in immediate awareness, the phenomena as encountered, precisely as they are encountered. Contemporary medical philosopher Kay Toombs explains that "the task" of phenomenology "is to elucidate and render explicit the taken-for-granted assumptions of everyday life and, particularly, to bring to the fore one's consciousness of the world. In rendering explicit the intentional structures of consciousness, phenomenological reflection discloses the meaning of experience" (Toombs 2001, 2).

This history of phenomenology highlights a paradox for U.S. medicine that could not be sharper. At the same time Flexner held up German medical education as the supreme model for U.S. medical training and research, Husserl, whom many consider the most important German philosopher of the twentieth century, exposed a fundamental problem at the core of this same European science. The U.S. medical system founded on European science did not commit Nazi-level abuses, but it did develop its own of "health care crisis" that in many ways mirrors Husserl's "European crisis."

To see this link between the contemporary "health care crisis" and Husserl's "European crisis" we have to look behind the headlines and sound bite coverage of today's health care crisis. The crisis in health care is about more than financial and administrative troubles. The crisis comes from deep and fundamental problems with the way health care is conceptualized. Indeed, the core problem for Flexner's medical science is the same as the one Husserl described for European science—the problem of naive objectivism. Medical science, under the Flexner model, so valorized "objective" medical facts that it lost sight of "subjective" and "human" experiences of illness and health care. In the years following the Flexner report, medicine gradually drifted toward "overspecialization; technicism; overprofessionalism; insensitivity to personal and sociocultural values; too narrow a construal of the doctor's role; too much 'curing' rather than 'caring'; not enough emphasis on prevention, patient participation, and patient education; too much economic incentive; a 'trade school' mentality; overmedicalization of everyday life; inhumane treatment of medical students; overwork by house staff; and deficiencies in verbal and nonverbal communication" (Pellegrino 1979, 9) This list of problems, first compiled by Pellegrino more than thirty years ago, all stem from the same fundamental flaw that sits at the heart of medicine—the loss of the human aspects of medical care.

As phenomenologist and medical philosopher Richard Zaner put it, medicine gradually became a kind of "applied biology." Flexner's biomedical vision was so successful that not only were clinicians impregnated with the fundamental truths of biology, but also they lost sight of much else. Zaner demonstrates by pointing to a typical case presentation from a medical journal: "A 22-year-old healthy nonsmoking man presented after coughing up a cup of bright-red blood. The initial history and physical examination were unrevealing. The chest roentgenogram, arterial blood gas levels, the complete blood count, indexes of coagulation, the platelet count, and the blood urea nitrogen concentration were all normal" (Zaner 1990, 303).

Zaner, looking at this case from the perspective of phenomenology, found himself in total befuddlement. The presentation gave no information about "who this man is, where he was, what he was doing, how he got to the hospital, or any other of a number of questions prompted simply by the fact that this 'case report' is not about rocks or twigs but a sick person" (1990, 303). Zaner asks, "How has it happened that people who are sick are 'presented' in this manner? Why is the history said to be 'unrevealing'?" He concluded that there can be only one response to this situation, a thorough "exploration into the heart of modern medicine, its educational emphasis, and its historical development" (1990, 303).

Many physicians trained in the Flexner model would agree that this case history does not tell the whole story, that the personhood of the patient matters, and that good bedside manner requires that the physician be aware of the whole individual. But, as physicians, they also would argue that their main job is to attend to the biology. Only with the turn to phenomenology and the experience of illness do the problems with this biomedical logic manifest themselves. With the turn to the phenomenology, it becomes clear that the challenge of being ill involves much more than biology alone. Whatever the biology involved, the patient's experience of illness, the patient's own unique form of suffering, must be understood in its own right. One cannot extrapolate from biology alone the person's unique situation or the unique form of struggle caused by the bodily impairment. To understand the illness, one has to turn to a different register beyond the mechanical and the animal. One must turn to human consciousness.

Pellegrino explained to his Flexner-trained colleagues that "illness is an altered state of existence arising out of an ontological assault on the humanity of the person who is ill" (Pellegrino 1982, 157). He identified four areas of compromise that befall the ill person. First, the person who is ill suffers a loss of freedom of action because of bodily impairment. Second, the person lacks the necessary information needed to make rational steps toward recovery. Third, the person loses some degree of autonomy and must increase his or her level of dependence on others. And, fourth, the person must transform his or her self-image consequent with the changed situation and increased vulnerability.

Together, these assaults on the ill constitute the "wounded humanity" of the patient. The patient's wounded humanity, instead of being a secondary aspect of the clinical encounter, is the bedrock of the healing relationship. "Healing," Pellegrino argued, "is a mutual act that aims to repair the defects created by the experience of illness" (Pellegrino 1982, 156). The only way the physician can legitimately enter into a healing relationship is through a phenomenological understanding of wounded humanity. Otherwise the physician has no hope of assisting the patient with the many compromises of illness. Tending to biological variables may be part of it, but only part. For Pellegrino, "if the professional does not consciously remedy the four deficiencies which impair the patient's expression of humanity, his 'profession' is inauthentic" (1979, 127). Indeed, "the moral authenticity of the healing act is thus measured by the fullness with which it remediates the afflicted state that illness represents" (1982, 157).

Medical philosophy was not alone in these insights. Interpretive approaches from medical anthropology and medical sociology reached similar conclusions. For example, in his influential book *The Illness Narratives: Suffering, Healing, and the Human Condition*, psychiatrist and medical anthropologist Arthur Kleinman also argued for a return to the illness experience. Based on twenty years of clinical research devoted to the chronic illness, Kleinman took the phenomenological wisdom the next step by documenting a series of "illness narratives" of chronic illness. In recording these stories, Kleinman made a basic distinction between "illness" and "disease" (Kleinman 1988, 3). *Illness* referred to the "innately human experience of symptoms and suffering," whereas *disease* was the clinical perspective of the problem. With the reign of Flexner's biomedical paradigm, disease was "reconfigured *only* as an alteration in biological structure or functioning" (1988, 5). But Kleinman found that biological variables alone could not explain the exacerbations and relative remissions of chronic illness. The only way to explain these ups and downs was through psychological and social variables.

Kleinman's illness narratives made a compelling case for the need to bridge the gap between patient and clinician. He argued for a meaning-centered medicine through which the clinician attends not only to patient's bodies but also to "1) empathic witnessing of the existential experience of suffering and 2) practical coping with the major psychosocial crises that constitute the menacing chronicity of that experience" (1988, 10). Like Pellegrino, Kleinman saw meaning-centered medicine as both more effective and more in tune with the central purpose of medicine. The perspective of chronic illness reveals that the purpose of medicine, what Kleinman called its "moral core," must be both control of disease *and* care for the illness experience (1988, 253).

For patients who have chronic illness (which increasingly is the vast majority of patients), "neither the interpretation of illness meanings nor the handling of deeply felt emotions within intimate personal relationships can be dismissed as peripheral tasks. They constitute, rather, the point of medicine. . . . Failure to address these issues is a fundamental flaw in the work of doctoring" (1988, 253). Kleinman argued that correcting the imbalance of medicine will require much more than "nice" or "artful" clinicians; it will require a basic reorientation of medical inquiry away from the Flexner model to include what he called "the human sciences of medicine": anthropology, sociology, psychology, history, philosophy, and literary studies (1988, 266). Without such a reorientation, medicine would remain cut off from its moral core, unable to meaningfully conceptualize illness experiences or provide truly effective healing.

Medical sociologists further documented the wisdom of Kleinman's insights. Kathy Charmaz, in her book *Good Days, Bad Days: The Self in Chronic Illness and Time*, used qualitative methods to understand how chronic illness not only affected bodies but also fundamentally reshaped people's sense of meaning and time (Charmaz 1991). And, in a particularly poignant example, Arthur Frank wrote a moving memoir that brought his sociological perspective to his own experiences with both cancer and a heart attack (Frank 1992). Frank found that the medical side of the experience, though helpful, was insufficient to cope with the task of working through the meaning of the illness for his life or the suffering that the disruption of illness created.

In a later book, *Wounded Storyteller: Body, Illness, and Ethics*, Frank pulled back from his own experiences to do qualitative research on a range of illness narratives (Frank 1995). He found that any serious illness, not just chronic illness, involves a loss of the previous life map that guided the ill person's life. As a result of this loss, "ill people have to learn to think differently" and the learning process involved occurs through storytelling (1995, 1). The ill learn to think differently by hearing themselves tell their stories, by absorbing other's reactions to these stories, and by experiencing their stories being shared. The stories of the ill work together to create a new life map, and the importance of developing this new life map means that the ill not only want to tell their stories, "they *need* to tell their stories, in order to construct new maps and new perceptions of their relationships to the world" (1995, 3).

Literature and medicine scholars added to the chorus reorienting medicine back to its humane core by a careful study of what physician and literary scholar Howard Brody calls the "stories of sickness" (Brody 2003). Representations of illness abound in literature, from classical accounts of plagues to the ubiquitous consumptive in Victorian novels to the multiple malignancies of contemporary literature and drama. These fictional accounts, as well as recent outpourings of nonfiction (biography and memoir), provide an ideal site for understanding the meaning of illness and healing (Hawkins and McEntyre 2000). Brody organized the many insights that come from reading this literature into a simultaneous appreciation of "storytelling as healing" and "healing as storytelling" (2003, 8).

Brody's understanding of *storytelling as healing* recognizes, in the tremendous diversity of illness stories, a common thread: "Suffering is produced and alleviated by the meaning that one attaches to one's experience. The primary human mechanism for attaching meaning to particular experiences is to tell stories about them" (2003, 13). These stories are much more than epiphenomena to the experience; in many ways, the stories determine the experience. For Brody, a good story is a central feature of what physicians call the "placebo effect" because a good story provides (1) an explanation consistent with the person's worldview, (2) a connection to a community of practitioners and concerned others who share this worldview, and (3) a sense of mastery and control over the experience (2003, 13).

Healing as storytelling flips the perspective from patient to clinician. It recognizes that clinicians not only hear stories but also spend much of their time telling stories. These stories, which Katherine Montgomery Hunter called "doctor stories," are similar to patient stories in that they use a narrative logic to understand and explain the person's difficulties (Hunter 1991). Medical science and the biological model usually provide the organizing metaphor, but applying this model to a unique individual going through a particular form of suffering or bodily difference requires taking up a narrative frame. The clinician listens to the patient's complaints and then inquires about other things according to his or her own frame of reference. "Pieced together with the patient's story, the answers to these questions are translated into pathophysicological concepts, and this augmented account of the patient's experience is edited and encoded in the chart" (1991, 6). An oral version is recounted in clinical rounds, and a translated version is given back to the patient. "Chillingly unrecognizable and 'scientific' as the resulting case may sound, it is a narrative" (1991, 7).

This medical reauthoring of the patient's story is not a problem in and of itself. As Hunter makes clear, this is exactly what in many cases patients come for—to have their story retold in a way that allows new and, it is to be hoped, beneficial strategies for healing. But close attention to the stories of illness, particularly recent memoirs and biographies, reveals that patient stories and doctor stories often do not work well together. Anne Hunsaker Hawkins refers to patient stories that conform or adapt to doctor stories as "medically syntonic" and those that do not as "medically dystonic" (Hawkins 1993, 21–22). Medically syntonic stories read like "religious testimonies, public professions of faith that are meant to bear witness to the truth and strengthen other believers by relating an experience of spiritual trial or conversion" (1993, 4). They are positive toward medicine and tell stories complimentary to medical treatment, which they see as generally helpful and appropriate.

Hawkins found that although medically syntonic testimonials were common in the 1960s and 1970s, by the 1980s memoirs and biographies had become much more dystonic. Trust in medicine and tolerance of hospital routines during this time move from the norm to "the exception," and published patient stories become dominated by angry and rejecting narratives. Angry narratives "expose and denounce atrocities in the way illness is treated in America today. These books testify to a medical system seen as out of control, dehumanized, and sometimes brutalizing" (1993, 6).

They are written from a sense of outrage and bitterness over medicine's too frequent failure to care for the ill. In a memoir of her mother's illness, Lee Ann Shreiber puts this anger and frustration succinctly: doctors are "specialists trained to intervene at moments of crisis, to cut, to radiate, to alter chemistry, then move on to the next patient. But why is there no place in this elaborate medical system for sustained care of the human being who continues to feel the effects of the doctors' knives and beams and chemicals?" (cited in Hawkins 1993, 6).

Hawkins found that many medically dystonic narratives are not so much angry as uninterested. These narratives tell stories of patients devoted to the pursuit of alternative healing approaches and treatment modalities. They often give physicians a role in their treatment attending to biochemical aspects of the problem, but this biochemical dimension is seen as less important than the more emotional and spiritual side—"the 'will to live' that has by now become a battle cry for many ill people" (1993, 9). These patient stories "fairly bristle with holistic and alternative therapies—therapies ranging from such relatively conventional practices as attention to diet and exercise, acupuncture, and visualization exercises to more unusual treatments: the use of quartz crystals, lucid dreams, and various naturopathic remedies" (1993, 9).

The Emergence of Narrative Medicine

This story of U.S. medicine brings us to the contemporary moment when the most insightful voices in medicine are calling for a narrative turn. The emergence of a broader medical scholarship since the time of Flexner provides the necessary background for understanding this narrative turn. Medicine is coming to understand, even if it has only partially corrected, the flaws of Flexner's overly biocentric approach. Narrative medicine is the umbrella term for a range of contemporary efforts to humanize medicine and counterbalance the many problems of Flexner's model. The term *narrative medicine* comes from Rita Charon, a Columbia University internist and literary scholar, who uses it to describe an approach to medicine that employs narrative approaches to augment scientific understandings of illness (Charon 2005, 261). Narrative medicine as Charon articulates it brings together insights from more inclusive medical models, such as Engel and Cassel, along with research and insights from phenom-enology, the humanities, and interpretive social sciences.

Narrative medicine practitioners use these resources to better under-stand the illness experience, "to recognize, absorb, interpret, and be moved by the stories of illness" (Charon 2006, vii). As Charon argues, when clinicians possess "narrative competency," they can enter the clinical set-ting with a nuanced capacity for "attentive listening . . . , adopting alien perspectives, following the narrative thread of the story of another, being curious about other people's motives and experiences, and tolerating the uncertainty of stories" (2005, 262). Doctors "*need* rigorous and disci-plined training" in narrative reading and writing not just for their own sake (helping deal with the strains and traumas of clinical work) but also "*for the sake of their practice*" (2005, 262). Without such narrative com-petency, clinicians lack the ability to fully understand their client's experi-ence of illness. For Charon and others in narrative medicine, narrative study is not a mere adornment to a doctor's medical training; it is a crucial and "basic science" that must be mastered for medical practice (Charon 2004, 863).

Narrative medicine helps students and clinicians gain this critical nar-rative competency through a variety of methods. Like literature and med-icine, narrative medicine emphasizes the parallels between acts of reading and acts of healing. In both reading and healing, the process begins with a story told by one person that another receives with the obligation to make sense of it. What the receiver does with the story will depend on the receiver's "absorptive powers, interpretive accuracy, characterlogical ten-dencies, and the bank of stories in the receiver's possession with which to compare or align this one" (Charon 2006, 108). For advocates of narra-tive medicine, "good readers make good doctors" because the fate of the received story depends on the preparation of the receiver (2006, 113). Narrative medicine prepares medical practitioners to receive these clinical stories through practice (by reading stories in clinical settings) and through theory (by using insights from humanities and interpretive social science—Kleinman's "human sciences of medicine") to better understand how clini-cal stories work.

In addition, narrative medicine advocates have been exploring the use of narrative writing for clinicians. Building on a long history of physician writers, Charon coined her version of this teaching approach the "Parallel Chart" (2006, 155). This device asks students and clinicians to write about their patients and about their own experiences in ordinary language. Writing down these experiences and reading them aloud with others counters the objectifying forces of the medical chart. It gives students and clinicians an opportunity to explore in detail their patient's experience of illness and their own personal and emotional reactions to clinical work. The Parallel Chart increases clinicians' capacity to process emotions and to appreciate unfolding life stories by increasing the skills of narrative representation and self-reflection.

Using these tools, narrative medicine creates clinicians who can stay with the emotional and personal complexities of illness without retreating into silent detachment or, worse, simply avoiding altogether the human aspects of health care. Because "sickness opens the door to knowledge of one's self and one's values," Charon explains, "the person who cares for the sick has to be prepared to midwife the life scrutiny that inevitably accompanies illness. We have to learn how to listen to the multiple registers of the body, the self, and the storyline and how to respond ethically and dutifully to what we hear" (2006, 182). Physicians must tend to this human part of health care as much as they tend to the animal part, "for the body will not bend to ministrations from someone who cannot recognize the self within it, the self exposed to the new light of day by virtue of ruptures in its surface of health" (2006, 182).

Conclusion

Medicine at its core is a deeply human practice. This simple statement explains why one hundred years after the Flexner report focused medical education, research, and practice on the animal part of medicine, on biological variables and biological interventions, medicine still struggles to find its balance. A medicine that leaves out the human dimensions of health care—the experience of patients, their desires, their preferences, and the social context in which these emerge—is a medicine in crisis. Individual physicians sometimes find a way to rise above their training to develop empathic and cultural skills, but all too often medicine has lost touch with the human aspects of health care and the clinical encounter. For a poignant example, consider Margaret Edson's Pulitzer Prize–winning play *Wit*.

Edson dramatically portrays how Flexnerian medicine can leave patients feeling like machines on an assembly line at times of their greatest vulnerability and deepest distress. And at a societal level, Edson shows how medicine that tends only to the body is a medicine that tilts ever more toward specialization, technical interventions, and unsustainable expenditures.

Each of us, even if we are currently temporarily able, is headed toward sickness and death. Both as individuals and as a culture, we must be wise in the face of our bodily impermanence. Our body alone cannot tell us how to make judgments and priorities in the face of its inevitable disease. We must make those kinds of judgments, and we can do this only if our humanness, our consciousness, and our life stories are let back into the research, education, and practice of health care. Narrative medicine builds on the wisdom of the past forty years of reform efforts in medicine to do just this. It draws from person-centered medicine, from the biopsychosocial model, and from humanities and cultural studies work in phenomenology, bioethics, narrative theory, and cultural and political difference. The emergence of narrative medicine is invaluable not only for medicine but also for the specialty of psychiatry. The hype and excitement of neuroscience, cognitive science, psychopharmacology, and cognitive therapy have begun to erode the human dimension of psychiatry and have left psychiatry vulnerable to losing its own balance. As I discuss in Chapter 4, when psychiatry embraces the wisdom of narrative medicine, this imbalance can be corrected. But before developing this argument for psychiatry, we must also look at the recently emergent role of narrative in psychotherapy.

CHAPTER THREE

Narrative Approaches to Psychotherapy

L EADING THINKERS IN PSYCHOTHERAPY, what we could consider the "other side" of psychiatry, have recently taken a narrative turn. And just as we had to tell a story to understand the rise of narrative medicine, we must also tell a story to understand the emergence of narrative approaches to psychotherapy. The story of psychotherapy I will tell, like many others before me, begins in the late nineteenth century with Sigmund Freud's creation of psychoanalysis. Freud's work established the very possibility of a "talking cure," and it was for many years the leading perspective in psychotherapy. Psychotherapists, however, were not content to follow Freud's lead, and over the course of the twentieth century psychotherapists created a vast array of competing psychotherapy alternatives. Only in the past few years have these competing forms of psychotherapy begun to cooperate, to communicate, and to integrate their ideas and practices.

The turn toward narrative in psychotherapy integration emerges as a response to this history of psychotherapeutic fragmentation and the recent desire for more integrated approaches. Narrative theory provides not only an open-minded alternative to contemporary psychotherapy turf wars but also a metatheoretical framework for integrating and making sense of the many available therapeutic options. The tremendous advantage of a narrative metatheoretical frame for psychotherapy integration is that it allows a renewed appreciation of the many forms of psychotherapy without having to choose one true and only correct method and without falling into an anything-goes relativism. It is precisely because narrative approaches answer this complex and subtle conceptual need that the narrative turn has been so important to contemporary psychotherapy and can be so valuable for contemporary psychiatry.

In this chapter, I provide a historical context for the emergence of narrative approaches to psychotherapy, review the basics of narrative theory that informs these approaches, and discuss a literary case example to bring out some of the main points of the discussion. I conclude with the two ways narrative theory has been used in psychotherapy practice: as the basis for a specific narrative psychotherapy and as a tool for psychotherapy integration. It is the second of these that is most critical for narrative psychiatry.

A Brief History of Psychotherapy

My plot line for the emergence of narrative approaches to psychotherapy is one that a psychoanalyst might call the "return of the repressed." Narrative insights were a key part of Freud's early work, but these insights were not valued or respected. Instead, they were repressed by Freud and a by century of struggle over specific psychotherapy models. This repression of narrative has started to thaw in recent times, allowing the return of narrative as a central concern for contemporary psychotherapy.

Psychiatrist James Phillips provides a nice analysis of Freud's early work to show that "narrative and narrative identity have been present in psychoanalysis from the beginning" (Phillips 1999, 28). But instead of developing this dimension of psychoanalysis, Freud lamented that his case histories sounded more like narrative fictions than hard science: "I have not always been a psychotherapist. Like other neuropathologists, I was trained to employ local diagnosis and electro-prognosis, and it still strikes me as strange that the case histories I write should read like short stories and that, as one might say, they lack the serious stamp of science" (Breuer and Freud 1955, 160). As this quotation reveals, Freud was ambivalent about (and at times embarrassed by) the narrative dimensions of his work. Despite his awareness of the importance of story in his clinical encounters, he never embraced a narrative theory of psychoanalysis. He remained manifestly attached throughout his career to the more sciencelike models he inherited from neuropathologists.

After Freud, psychotherapy goes through a century of competing models—what could be called the "battle of the brands"—which further downplays the role of narrative in psychotherapy. In the battle of the brands, the emphasis was the specific models, not the possibility that all therapies work through narrative storytelling.

Psychoanalysis begins the battle of the brands by rapidly splintering itself into a host of psychotherapy alternatives. Psychoanalysis initially divided around Freud's drive theory—which emphasized unconscious libidinal and aggressive drives as the primary motive for action. Early splits from Freud's classical drive theory came from Alfred Adler and Carl Jung. Later on, from the 1940s to the 1970s, additional splits included ego psychologists (who argued that drive theory must be extended to include relative autonomy of ego functions) and Lacanians (who underscored the importance of language for the functioning of the unconscious). From the 1970s to the 1990s, further splits in psychoanalysis included the object-relations theorists (who emphasized the importance of human motives for attachment) and the relational school (who focused on the importance of ongoing relatedness as the fundamental building block of mental life).

This splintering of psychoanalysis into different schools was just the beginning of the growth of psychotherapy alternatives. Much of the further splintering outside psychoanalysis was around the question of science in psychotherapy. Behavioral psychologists, unhappy with any of the versions of psychoanalysis, consistently attacked the Freudian corpus as not being sufficiently scientific. J. B. Watson initiated the attack in 1913 when he published a behaviorist manifesto in the *Psychological Review*: "Psychology as the behaviorist views it is a purely objective branch of natural science. Its theoretical goal is the prediction and control of behavior. Introspection forms no essential part of its methods, nor is the scientific value of its data dependent upon the readiness with which they lend themselves to interpretation in terms of consciousness" (Watson 1913, 158). For Watson and the early behaviorists (such as Ivan Pavlov, Joseph Wolpe, and B. F. Skinner), psychology was an unambiguous branch of natural science, and as such it could be nothing like psychoanalysis. Instead of being mentalist, subjective, and partially deterministic, it must be materialistic, objective, and fully deterministic (Fishman and Franks 1992, 162).

Throughout the 1950s and 1960s, behavioral therapists used these principles along with the concepts of learning theory to develop an extensive behavioral therapy alternative to psychoanalysis. But by the 1970s behavioral therapy itself began to splinter into different submovements.

These different behaviorist therapies divided along a continuum of approaches that were more or less open to the inclusion of unobservable cognitive processes. At one end of the spectrum and most true to B. F. Skinner's early operant conditioning models was applied behavioral analysis, which relied on the assumption that behavior was function of consequences. These behavioral therapists intervened through procedures (like reinforcement, extinction, and stimulus control) that altered the relationship between behavior and consequences without concern for cognitive or mentalist variables. At the other end of the spectrum, cognitive behavioral therapists stood on the shoulders of the cognitive revolution in psychology to argue that learned cognitive processes mediate behavioral response. For cognitive behaviorists, impaired (or dysfunctional) cognition creates mental problems, and therapy works through uncovering and correcting these cognitive distortions.

During the same time period that behavioral therapy was establishing itself, a group of humanistic psychologists came on the scene who were also concerned with the science question in psychoanalysis. For humanistic psychologists, the problem with psychoanalysis was not that it was insufficiently scientific (as the behaviorists had claimed) but just the opposite. Psychoanalysis relied too heavily on the logics of science. Humanistic psychologists rejected both the ambiguous scientism of psychoanalysis and the radical scientism of behaviorism by arguing that psychology was not a natural science but a human study. Proponents of humanistic psychology, often described as psychology's "third force," formed the American Association for Humanistic Psychology in 1962 and by 1970 had founded a subdivision within the American Psychological Association. At the same time, humanistic psychologists also began an informal association with the Esalen Institute, in Big Sur, California, which solidified their connections within the broader human potential movement and youth counterculture.

The connection with the human potential movement provides a window on a key aspect of humanistic psychology: it was a reaction to not just the mechanistic scientism of psychology but also to deeper yearnings and currents in the culture at large. For humanistic psychologists, "the aridity of modern psychological theory and its picture of man was in itself symptomatic of a deadening alienation and a dehumanization that had badly infected the entire social fabric" (Shaffer 1978, 6). As an antidote to the alienating effects of psychoanalytic and behavioral psychotherapy, humanistic psychotherapy emphasized four central themes:

1. A phenomenological approach that views the client as the expert of his or her own experience
2. A deep commitment to human capacities for self-growth and actualization
3. A belief in the human agency as the final arbitrator of choice and self-determination
4. A person-centered focus that includes a deep respect for the uniqueness of each individual (Rice and Greenberg 1992, 198–99)

Most humanistic psychotherapists accepted these four central themes, but, alas, they also quickly divided into variety of competing approaches. These included client-centered psychotherapy developed by Carl Rogers, Gestalt psychotherapy developed by Fritz Perls, and existential psychotherapy developed by Ludwig Binswanger and Medard Boss.

Beyond the emergence of multiple psychoanalytic, behaviorist, and humanistic alternatives, the world of psychotherapy splintered even further in the last quarter of the twentieth century. Additional alternatives that gained ground in the 1970s and 1980s included a variety of family therapies, group therapies, interpersonal therapies, feminist therapies, creative therapies, and spiritual therapies, just to name a few. This proliferation has continued up to the current moment, with more than four hundred competing systems of psychotherapy now being practiced (Corsini and Wedding 2005, 9).

The most interesting thinking in psychotherapy today involves the question of how to understand the meaning of this psychotherapeutic diversity and how to move beyond a century of competing psychotherapeutic brands. Contemporary researchers and theorists of psychotherapy have responded to psychotherapeutic diversity with two main strategies. Some have put their faith in science as the arbitrator between psychotherapies—only this time using the science of outcome studies rather than behavioral science. Others are rethinking the very goals and ideals of modern science as applied to psychotherapy from a postmodern perspective. Interestingly, both of these responses to psychotherapeutic diversity have yielded advocates for a broadly integrative psychotherapy that can be understood through the tools of narrative theory.

The first strategy, outcome studies, rests on the idea that science might still sort out different models through the use of outcome studies to determine which approaches work best. The most well-known version of this research, empirically supported therapies (EST), uses clinical trials methodology and treatment manuals to pair specific treatments with specific disorders. The clinical trials approach has produced some compelling results, such as the value of exposure techniques for anxiety and behavioral techniques for certain sexual problems like the "pause technique" for premature ejaculation (Ogles, Anderson, and Lunnen 1999, 213). But, as Michael Lambert explained in his 2007 presidential address to the Society for Psychotherapy Research, this approach has also "stirred widespread debate about the wisdom of assuming that effective treatments can be so simply defined and delivered" (Lambert 2007, 1).

Lambert and other scientifically minded critics of EST also rely on outcome studies to argue that the battle of the brands is unlikely to be fruitful. They point to a less well-known but equally important tradition of psychotherapy research that uses meta-analysis comparisons. These outcome studies have yielded two major findings. The first is that psychotherapy works. Researchers estimate that more than two-thirds of patients in psychotherapy make improvements (Lambert 2007; Lambert and Bergin 1994). The second is no specific approach to psychotherapy is superior. Decades of meta-analysis reviews find that alternative approaches to psychotherapy are all *equally effective* (Luborsky, Singer, and Luborsky 1975; Luborsky et al. 2002; Wampold 2001, 2006).

The psychotherapeutic research community lovingly refers to this second finding as the "Dodo bird verdict." The name is based on a classic paper by Saul Rosenzweig that contained a prophetic epigraph from *Alice in Wonderland*: "At last, Dodo said, everybody has won and all must have prizes" (Rosenzweig 1936). The remarkable consistency of the Dodo bird verdict in meta-analysis studies suggests that the positive effects of therapy have relatively little to do with the specific interventions of therapist and come largely from nonspecific factors. In a widely referenced work, Lambert carried the Dodo bird verdict to the next step. He used the extensive psychotherapy research database to estimate the relative percentages of the elements accounting for client improvement (Lambert 1992). He concluded that 40 percent of change comes from client personal resources (both psychological and environmental), 30 percent from common features of therapists (such as empathy, warmth, acceptance, and encouragement of risk taking), and 15 percent from client trust and expectation (sometimes called placebo). That left only 15 percent of change coming from the therapist's specific techniques and theoretical models.

These findings are not the last word in psychotherapy research. Both EST and the Dodo bird verdict remain controversial, and outcome studies of psychotherapy will continue for some time.[1] Nonetheless, the Dodo has been highly influential, and it has many supporters in the psychotherapy community (Duncan 2002a). For these supporters, the Dodo bird verdict means that the process of setting up a therapeutic relationship with a quality therapist is much more important than the content of the therapist's specific models and theories. It also means that a variety of theoretical models can be used to understand, cope with, and ameliorate difficult emotional states.[2] In the classic words of Rosenzweig: "Whether the therapist talks in terms of psychoanalysis or Christian Science is . . . relatively unimportant as compared with the formal consistency with which the doctrine employed is adhered to, for by virtue of this consistency the patient receives a schema for achieving some sort and degree of personality organization" (Rosenzweig 1936, 413–15).

Psychiatrist Jerome Frank beautifully articulated similar insights in *Persuasion and Healing: A Comparative Study of Psychotherapy* (third edition, coauthored by Julia Frank): "[It] is not that technique is irrelevant to outcome. Rather, . . . the success of all techniques depends on the patient's sense of alliance with an actual or symbolic healer. This position implies that ideally therapists should select for each patient the therapy that accords, or can be brought into accord, with the patient's personal characteristics and view of the problem. Also implied is that therapists should seek to learn as many approaches as they find congenial and convincing. Creating a good therapeutic match may involve both educating the patient about the therapist's conceptual scheme and, if necessary, modifying the scheme to take into account the concepts the patient brings to therapy" (Frank and Frank 1991, xv). From this perspective we can see that engagement in a psychotherapeutic relationship becomes a care and practice of the self. It is not an exercise in absolute relativism or an objective discovery of a universally true self. It is a collaborative partnership that helps develop and crystallize a certain kind of subjectivity.

Jerome Frank was not a postmodernist, but his insights start to sound like the writings of postmodern theory—which is the second important way (beyond outcome studies) psychotherapists have tried to make sense of the proliferating options for psychotherapy. Postmodern psychotherapy theorists have taken advantage of the wealth of resources in theoretical humanities to help make sense of psychotherapeutic diversity.[3] Postmodern theory in the humanities is a collection of writings coming first from Continental philosophers—such as Michel Foucault, Jacques Derrida, and Luce Irigaray—and later extended into the U.S. academy by writers like Richard Rorty, Judith Butler, and Gayatri Spivak. These writers have in common a deep appreciation of the way language shapes meaning and perception and the ways that power relations shape language. Postmodern theories provide valuable resources for appreciating psychotherapeutic diversity—as they do for multicultural diversity more broadly—because postmodern theories understand that different linguistic systems and cultural practices will necessarily interpret the world and interact with the world in different ways (Lewis 2006b).

From a postmodern perspective, different ways of engaging psychotherapy do not map out along a hierarchical modern science grid of true/good theories at the top and false/bad theories at the bottom. Instead, each different way of engaging psychotherapy has its own truths and its own value priorities built into it. For example, cognitive behavioral therapy is not understood from a postmodern logic as truer and therefore universally better than relational psychoanalysis. Rather, cognitive behavioral psychotherapy will be informative about and good for some things (clarifying cognitive distortions) and relational psychoanalysis informative about and good for other things (gaining insight into the emotional dynamics of relations). From a postmodern perspective, whether one picks cognitive behavioral therapy or relational psychoanalysis will depend partly on questions of truth (what kind of knowledge claims seem legitimate to you) and partly on questions of goals, values, and esthetics.

This postmodern perspective fits well with one of the most profound aspects of Rosenzweig's original Dodo bird reference. Rosenzwieg, an avid fan of literature, chose the Dodo bird epigraph carefully to articulate his insights on psychotherapeutic diversity (Duncan 2002b, 20). In the section from *Alice in Wonderland* he selects, Lewis Carroll tells the story of a group of animals who were soaked by Alice's tears. The Dodo bird, in order to help the animals dry off, starts them in a "caucus-race." It's informative to look closely at this section.

> First it [the Dodo bird] marked out a race-course, in a sort of a circle ("the exact shape does not matter," it said) and then all the party were placed along the course, here and there. There was no "one, two, three, and away," but they began running when they liked, and left off when they liked, so that it was not easy to know when the race was over. However, when they had been running half an hour or so, and were quite dry again, the Dodo suddenly called out "The race is over!" and they all crowded around it, panting, and asking, "But who has won?"
>
> This question the Dodo could not answer without a great deal of thought, and it sat for a long time with one finger pressed upon its forehead (the position in which you usually see Shakespeare, in the pictures of him), while the rest waited in silence. At last the Dodo said, "Everybody has won and all must have prizes." (Carroll 1992, 34–35)

As this passage makes clear, the Dodo bird's caucus race is not a race like other races. The animals do not start at the same place (or even at the same time), nor do they end at the same place.

Because the race was so unusual, the verdict that "everybody has won" does not mean that the race was a tie. It means that the animals' many different individual races are incommensurable, or not easily comparable, with each other (an idea at the heart of postmodern theory).[4] No one can say who ran the best race because they all ran different races. Which race is "best" depends on the goals of the runner. Do you want to start here or there? Now or later? Do you want to end up here or there? Because all the animals start at different places and end up at different places, not to mention that they all got more or less dry, the only possible answer to who won is "It depends." Ingeniously, the Dodo bird translates "It depends" into "Everybody has won!" From a postmodern perspective, the situation with psychotherapies is similar. Psychotherapeutic approaches are largely incomparable with each other because they pick different kinds of problems and they work toward different goals. The answer to the question of "Who wins" has a great deal to do with goals of therapy and the preferences of the client.

These insights on psychotherapeutic diversity coming from both outcome research and postmodern theory help us conclude our history of psychotherapy and understand the zeitgeist of psychotherapy today. Most psychotherapists today may not be particularly preoccupied with outcome research or postmodern theory, but they do approach their clinical work in a broadly open-minded way that is consistent with both these scholarships. Surveys of psychotherapists have found that 68 percent of therapists claim to be eclectic, with the average therapist using a combination of four different models (Jensen, Bergin, and Greaves 1990). Other studies have found that up to 90 percent of therapists embraced several therapeutic orientations (Norcross, Karpiak, and Santoro 2005). These studies suggest that most practicing psychotherapists mix and match theories and interventions depending on the situation. They call what they do "psychotherapy" or just "therapy" (rather than give it labels like cognitive behavioral, or interpersonal, or psychodynamic), and they easily combine psychoanalytic-oriented approaches with behavioral desensitizing techniques and humanistic unconditional positive regard (just to name a few).

Over the past several years, the informal eclecticism of most psychotherapists has grown into more formal approaches. Under the banner of "psychotherapy integration," eclectically minded therapists now have a journal (*Journal of Psychotherapy Integration*) and a professional society (Society for the Exploration of Psychotherapy Integration). Factors beyond the Dodo bird verdict and the rise of postmodern theories pushing toward increased psychotherapy integration include pressures from third-party payers, the fact that many of the founders of psychotherapy have now died and left a more open-minded succeeding generation, and a general trend in the broader culture toward cosmopolitanism and multicultural acceptance of diversity (Gold and Stricker 2006, 5). Bringing these factors together, psychologists Gold and Stricker may be premature in concluding that "the age of psychotherapeutic turf wars has ended," but they are certainly correct that there is a general trend within psychotherapy toward increasing integration and mutual learning (2006, 4).

Narrative approaches to psychotherapy integration can be especially helpful at this historical moment because narrative theory provides a metatheoretical orientation from which to understand human experience and to practice psychotherapy. Narrative allows psychotherapists to understand the common factors within psychotherapy and to appreciate the diversity of psychotherapeutic models without attempting to close these differences down (Angus and McLeod 2004; Hoshmand 2000; Richert 2006). In addition, narrative provides a theoretical frame for understanding how a range of different approaches, including different approaches to eclecticism and integration, might all be helpful in a therapeutic setting. At the same time, narrative approaches allow therapists to stay in touch with and informed by the data of research. Narrative can pay attention to compelling EST research, such as the importance of exposure techniques for anxiety problems, without insisting that these data are the last or the only word in therapeutic decision making.[5] In short, narrative approaches to psychotherapy integration have the flexibility to stay true to the wisdom of the Dodo bird, and they can also take advantage of useful findings from EST research.

This emergence of narrative psychotherapy integration brings our history of psychotherapy back full circle. More than a hundred years after Freud introduced "talking therapy," psychotherapy has returned to its early appreciation of the similarity between case histories and narrative stories.

Narrative Theory

To go further in our consideration of the role of narrative for psychotherapy, we must step back from our historical work and spend some time with the basics of narrative theory. The focus of this book does not allow me to go into tremendous detail of narrative theory, but we cannot skip the basics. Without grounding in the key features of narrative, many of the issues I discuss in later chapters will remain counterintuitive.

A central idea for understanding narrative theory begins with a distinction between *content* and *form*. Most of us, in our everyday reading and listening, read and listen for content. We focus our attention on the particular events being narrated. We look at what the author is telling us: what is the story, what is the news, what has happened? Our focus on content pays little attention to the form, or how the author tells the story. For narrative scholars, however, the content of a story or text is only the beginning. Narrative scholars approach a story with a series of additional questions about the form. They want to know how a story conveyed its meaning, through what specific authorial choices. And they want to know how the author structured the text so that it has the impact that it does.

Narrative scholars articulate these elements of narrative form in a variety of ways, and it would take an entire treatise on narrative theory to sort them out. But for our purposes, narrative physician Abraham Verghese's emphasis on *metaphor, plot,* and *character* as the elements of narrative most important for clinical settings is a good place to start. Verghese's emphasis on these three elements of narrative parallels the much more extensive and detailed narrative philosophy of Paul Ricoeur. In the sections that follow, I stand particularly on the shoulders of Ricoeur's work to provide an overview of narrative theory as relevant to narrative psychotherapy. After discussing the elements of metaphor, plot, and character, I discuss a literary example that not only shows how metaphor and plot come together in narrative identity but also adds the critical concept of *point of view* to the list of the elements of narrative.

METAPHOR

The stories people tell are rich with metaphor. Consider this snippet of a story from clinical life: "My boss looked at me yesterday like I was piece of garbage. He sees me as used up, something to discard and throw away. Talking to him leaves me feeling like shit. I'm worthless, my life is meaningless." This short snippet has at least four metaphors. The person compares himself or herself to garbage, shit, monetary value, and a literary text. Common sense would tell us that these kinds of metaphors have little importance. Metaphor in most people's minds may embellish or add ornamentation to the content of a story, but it does little else. From this commonsense perspective, the person behind the snippet feels bad and believes the boss doesn't value him or her. End of meaning. The literal paraphrase is all you need.

But for influential literary theorists, such as I. A. Richards, for a number of philosophers, particularly Max Black, Mary Hesse, Paul Ricoeur, and Mark Johnson, and increasingly for cognitive scientists like George Lakoff, metaphor has a much larger function. In their book *Metaphors We Live By*, Lakoff and Johnson put it most succinctly: "Metaphor is not just a matter of language, that is, of mere words. . . . On the contrary, human thought processes are largely metaphorical" (Lakoff and Johnson

1980, 6). Throughout their book, Lakoff and Johnson argue that metaphor is a pervasive aspect of human life, not just in the words that we use but also in our very concepts. "Our ordinary conceptual system, in terms of which we both think and act, is fundamentally metaphorical in nature" (1980, 3). By shaping our concepts, metaphor structures the way we perceive the world, what we experience, how we relate to other people, and the choices we make.

Metaphor works by allowing us to understand and experience one thing in terms of something else. Hesse uses the example, borrowed from Black, of "man is a wolf" (Hesse 2000, 351). Hesse explains that the metaphor works because it transfers ideas and associations from one term to the other. The metaphor selects, accentuates, and backgrounds aspects of two systems of ideas so that they come to be seen as similar. As Hesse explains, "Men are seen to be more like wolves after the wolf metaphor is used, and wolves seem to be more human" (2000, 351). Through metaphor the two terms, or, more precisely, the two systems of terms, interact with and adapt to each other. Understanding metaphor in this way changes standard ideas about truth and objectivity and allows us to sidestep the usual binary traps between relativism (anything goes) and realism (there is only one correct or true way to describe the world). When we understand language as a mediator between our concepts and the world, it no longer makes sense to think in these terms.[6]

As Ricoeur put it, we can let our notions of universal truth (or single objective truth) give way to ideas about "metaphorical truths" (Ricoeur 1977, 247). The many metaphors that shape our concepts and our perception allow us to see and experience the world in a particular ways. Ricoeur calls these many ways of perceiving the world "metaphorical *truths*" to emphasize that the metaphorical process is not just about words and concepts. Metaphor does allow us to understand something real, or true, about the world. But that reality is not absolute, and it is always in tension with other metaphorical options for understanding something equally real about the world. This tension is ultimately irreducible because when we change metaphors we change which aspects of the world we select, accentuate, and background.

Metaphor therefore allows us to make meaning, and it shapes our meaning at the same time. It enables us and constrains us simultaneously. To appreciate this aspect of metaphor, Ricoeur argues that it helps to remember that the verb "is," which holds a metaphor together, works as a relative term, not an absolute term. The metaphor "man *is* a wolf," Ricoeur poetically argues, "preserves the 'is not' within the 'is' " (1977, 249). Man, in this metaphorical frame, is both like a wolf and is not like a wolf. The "is" and the "is not" are both preserved in the metaphor.

PLOT

Plot works like metaphor in that plot also orders our experience and gives form to our narratives. Plot and the process of emplotment add to metaphor two key dimensions: (1) plot brings together what would otherwise be separate and heterogeneous elements, and (2) plot organizes our temporal perception—our understanding and experience of time.

The first critical function of plot for narrative is that it creates a narrative synthesis between multiple elements and events and brings them together into a single story. Plot allows an intelligible connection to be made between the elements of the story. And plot creates a synthesis between elements that are otherwise incongruous or heterogeneous—events that do not seem to fit together. With this function of plot it possible to have understandable stories with wildly diverse and disparate parts. For example, human desires, human rationality, human purpose, human agency, unconscious motives, unintended circumstances, unplanned accidents, other peoples' desires and rationality, other peoples' unconscious motives, material force, natural laws, divine intervention, discoveries, nightmares, historical chance, prejudice, the hand of God, economic downturns, failures of communication, contemporary styles and fashions, the effects of collaboration and conflict, grassroots organizing, spiritual conversion, the weather, technological capacity, and cell phones (just to name a few) are all easily brought together through the process of emplotment. Without a plot, we have no way to make sense of such wildly diverse phenomena.

In addition, plot is essential for human meaning because it configures the multiple elements of narrative into a temporal order that is crucial for our experience of time. Without plot to give us a temporal order, we cannot make sense of time. The temporal order of plot is of two sorts. First, each plot is composed of a series of discrete incidents, of theoretically infinite *nows*. Second, each plot takes these infinite nows, proceeding one after another in succession, and organizes them into a humanly manageable experience. As Ricoeur points out, without plot, time understood as a series of nows, what we could call "clock time," is an abstraction that cannot be experienced. The gap between clock time and the experience of "human time" comes from a well-known paradox: "The future is not yet, the past is no longer, and the present does not remain" (Ricoeur 1984, 7). Because clock time is fleeting, when we are asked to describe it, we are baffled.

Ricoeur finds a phenomenological solution to the riddle of human time in Saint Augustine's "thesis of the threefold present" (1984, 10). Augustine argued that present, past, and future exist simultaneously in the human mind through a coming together in a plural, or threefold, present. This threefold present includes the present moment plus *memory* and *expectation*. Memory recalls the past, and expectation, in an analogous way, looks toward the future. The present, in other words, contains our memory of the past and our expectation of future events. Critically, this threefold present highlights a parallel between the experience of time and the structure of narrative plots. Plot, like human time, is organized in a temporal order composed of three parts: beginning, middle, and end. The three parts of plot work like Augustine's threefold present. Ricoeur's key insight from this analysis of time and plot is that only through narrative plots are we able configure our otherwise confused, unformed, and mute temporal experience.

Ricoeur sees the relation between time and plot as a two-way phenomenon: time becomes human time when it is organized by plot, and, conversely, plot is meaningful because it portrays the features of temporal experience. Ricoeur admits that his conclusion is "undeniably circular," but he argues that this circularity is not in itself a problem: the circle of plot and time he explains is "not a vicious, but a healthy circle" (1984, 3). Emplotment, from this perspective, can be seen as a kind of prosthetic device. It does not solve the riddle of time so much as it allows us to keep going without a solution. The riddle of time is an inconclusive rumination to which the process of emplotment alone can respond: "Emplotment . . . replies to the speculative aporia [of time] with a poetic making of something capable, certainly, of clarifying the aporia . . . , but not of resolving it theoretically" (1984, 6).

The concept of character in literature brings us into contemporary controversies over the more basic concepts of self and identity. The controversy around what it means to be a self involves a deep tension between essentialist and nonessentialist approaches. On the one hand, essentialist notions of identity tell us that we have a fixed personality, perhaps biologically stamped, that is authentically ours and that is at the core of our being. This "true self" or "core self" may be distorted or covered over, but it is nonetheless there for the discovery if we apply ourselves patiently and persistently to the task. On the other hand, a variety of nonessentialist critiques have deconstructed this ideal of identity and its notion of an integral, originary, and unified self. Nonessentialist approaches argue instead for a much more social and linguistically constructed understanding of self and identity. This critique has been comprehensively advanced by Continental philosophers like Roland Barthes, Jacques Derrida, and Michel Foucault and by psychoanalytic writers working in the tradition of Jacques Lacan politically inflected through cultural studies and feminism.

One of the most productive ways to navigate the tension between essentialist and nonessentialist understandings of identity has been to draw a comparison between identity in life and character in fiction. Instead of adopting a linear logic that understands identity as a concept more fundamental to character, this approach uses a comparative logic to argue that we understand ourselves the same way we understand characters. Ricoeur calls this approach to identity "narrative identity," and the basic idea is critical to understanding the turn to narrative in psychology and psychotherapy. As Ricoeur puts it, "Fiction, in particular narrative fiction, is an irreducible dimension of self-understanding . . . fiction is only completed in life and life can be understood only through the stories that we tell about it" (Ricoeur 1991b, 30). Self-understanding, in this account, is an interpretive event and narrative is the privileged form for this interpretation: "A life story [is] a fictional history or, if one prefers, a historical fiction, interweaving the historiographic style of biographies with the novelistic style of imaginary autobiographies" (Ricoeur 1992, 114).

Literary theorist Peter Brooks sums up this idea up beautifully in his book *Reading for the Plot: Design and Intention in Narrative*: "Our lives are ceaselessly intertwined with narrative, with the stories that we tell and hear told, those we dream or imagine or would like to tell, all of which are reworked in that story of our own interrupted monologue. We live immersed in narrative, recounting and reassessing the meaning of our past actions, anticipating the outcome of our future projects, situating ourselves ant the intersection of several stories not yet completed" (Brooks 1984, 3). This kind of narrative approach to identity allows us to navigate the tension between essentialist and nonessentialist identities because narrative identity allows for continuity over time, a relative stability of self, without implying a substantial or essentialist core to this stability. The stability of our narrative interpretations comes not from an individual essence but from the weight of the cultural stories with which we are surrounded.

Aspects of our biological constitution such as our height or our personality dispositions will contribute to these stories, but they do not determine the stories. Body size, for example, can mean many things in different cultural settings. The cultural narratives in which we live help us organize the many variables that go into our identities and allow us to tell a story of self that escapes the two poles of random change and absolute fixity. In this way, a narrative identity is also a cultural identification. Our identifications may seem original, but we narrate them with the resources of history, language, and culture.

Cultural theorist Stuart Hall argues that identity is a "process of becoming rather than being: not 'who we are' or 'where we came from,' so much as what we might become, how we have been represented and how that bears on how we might represent ourselves" (Hall 1996, 4). Culturally narrated identities, Hall argues, involve "not the so-called return to roots, but a coming-to-terms with our 'routes'" (1996, 4). They involve asking ourselves which routes have we taken, how have those routes affected us, and what new routes might we choose ahead. This coming to terms with routes, although it involves a fictional use of cultural narratives, in no way undermines the material or political efficacy of identity, nor does it undermine a genuine sense of belonging that can come from a well-narrated self.

A LITERARY EXAMPLE

For an illustration of how metaphor and plot come together in narrative identity, consider the following literary example. Claire Messud's novel *The Emperor's Children* contains a scene in which two friends from college,

Danielle and Marina, plan on having dinner together. Both friends are in their early thirties; Danielle lives alone, and Marina lives with her parents. The dinner will be at Marina's house, but Danielle arrives first, which leaves her spending several minutes alone with Marina's parents. The situation makes Danielle feel awkward and uncomfortable. Here's the description of the scene: "Danielle . . . felt like a teenager, as she used to feel in the kitchen of her parents house in Columbus, before the divorce of course, and she was suddenly, powerfully, aware of the profound oddity of Marina's present life. A life arrested at, or at least returned to, childhood. Danielle couldn't imagine eating nightly with her parents, not only because they now lived in different states and didn't speak to each other, but because she was entering the fourth decade of life and hadn't been through the wearying rigmarole of family life for anything more than an almost supportable day since she was seventeen and had gone off to college" (Messud 2006, 46).

In this example, Danielle uses the *metaphor* of childhood to organize her understanding of Marina's life. Through the childhood metaphor Danielle perceives Marina's adult life as "arrested at, or at least returned to, childhood." Were Danielle to tell the story of Marina's life, she would pick out events from Marina's past that lead up to this moment. Perhaps she would recall a difficulty Marina had committing to relationships, or a series of immature reactions to authority figures, or a perhaps several examples of her being dreamy and irresponsible. These diverse elements would come together in a *plot* that leads to the present moment of Marina as trapped in childhood. The story would not only make sense of the past and the present and provide a *narrative identity* for Marina but also provide clear direction for the future. Marina must "grow up." She must leave her parents' home, get a job, marry, have children (or at least make steps in these directions).

This example makes clear the importance of adding "point of view" to our previous discussion of metaphor, plot, and character. Narratives tell a story from a particular perspective. Even if an author uses the omniscient point of view, that is still not a story from nowhere; it remains a story told by an author who has a particular take on the events he or she selects and frames. In the example from *The Emperor's Children*, we learn about Marina's life from Danielle's point of view. This passage does not tell us whether Marina would see herself as stuck in childhood; it tells us only that Danielle sees her this way. But, as it turns out, a little further on in the story, we learn that Marina has similar feelings about herself, and the perspective has left her unhappy and anxious about her life and about her worth as a person.

Not only this, as the novel proceeds, Marina's discontent with her childish life leads her into a whirlwind romance and a decision to marry an older magazine editor after they have been going out for a few weeks. In the process, Marina gains in rapid succession not only a husband but also a job (as she joins the editorial staff of the magazine). This rapid marriage and entrance into the job market effectively disrupt the childhood metaphor. But unfortunately Marina's judgments turn out to have been potentially premature, as the magazine quickly fails and the relationship falters. By the end of the novel, we do not know whether Marina's relationship will work, but Messud leaves her readers feeling skeptical.

Two Roles for Narrative Theory in Psychotherapy

Narrative theory has been helpful for psychotherapy in two ways. First, narrative theory has been inspirational for a specific form of psychotherapy known as "narrative psychotherapy." Second, and most critical for narrative psychiatry, narrative theory is an ideal conceptual tool for integrative approaches to psychotherapy. Our literary example from *The Emperor's Children* can help us understand these two ways narrative theory is helpful for psychotherapy.

NARRATIVE PSYCHOTHERAPY

Starting with narrative therapy as a specific form of psychotherapy, most of the work here has been inspired by Michael White and David Epston (White 2007; White and Epston 1990). Narrative psychotherapy begins with the client and therapist joining together for a collaborative deconstruction of the presenting story by carefully and lovingly pulling the story apart. Narrative psychotherapy begins this way because the basic idea is that the client comes to therapy with "broken" or "problematic" stories. These stories are constructed of metaphors, plots, narrative identifications, and points of view that disempower the person, overly limit his or her options, and are at the heart of his or her "psychological problems."

If we imagine that Marina decided on a narrative psychotherapy option, she and her narrative psychotherapist would start by looking together for gaps and breaks in her story. They would look for inconsistencies, for left-out information, for overly emphasized events, and for metaphors and plots that ground the assumptions of her story. Finding these kinds of gaps and inessential authorial choices would help Marina appreciate that her presenting story is not an absolute necessity for her self-understanding and that other stories could be told. Marina and the therapist would then work together to find a new story that would help Marina reauthor her past and present and expand her future options in desirable ways.

Unlike other psychotherapy options, narrative psychotherapy would be less likely to rely on therapeutic jargon and pretold story frames—such as are more common in psychoanalytic therapy, cognitive therapy, interpersonal therapy, or feminist therapy. Instead of using prerehearsed therapeutic frames, narrative psychotherapy would stay as close as possible to the language of everyday meaning and folk psychology. In addition, narrative psychotherapy, more than most other therapy options, tends to be conscious of cultural power dynamics and the way that people's problems often have to do with internalized hierarchies that they have adopted from mainstream culture.

In Marina's case, the metaphor of "childhood" provides a good example of the kinds of cultural power dynamics that she and a narrative psychotherapist might address. Marina lives in an elite, and still deeply patriarchal, culture in which "autonomy" and "independence" are given priority over "connection" and "interdependence." These cultural norms are loaded into the meaning of the "childhood" metaphor, and if a person is not autonomous and independent, he or she will likely be labeled negatively with the metaphor. A common way this happens is to say someone is "childish." This prejudice easily slides into "childism," in which negative attitudes become a deep-seated prejudice (Adams 2000; Pierce and Allen 1975). If Marina lived in a different culture, or if she thought through these values preferences in the context of narrative therapy, she might feel very different about her current life and what it means to live at home. In narrative therapy, Marina and the therapist would likely look for aspects of Marina's life, what narrative therapists call "unique outcomes," that go against the grain of the childhood metaphor. They would look at the many ways that Marina's life is very different from the life of a child, and they would deconstruct the wisdom of "childism" and the cultural insistence on norms of autonomy and independence.

Marina and her narrative therapist would question together whether these values preferences are absolute. Do they necessarily lead to a contented life, and are there examples in which people have followed these goals and ended up discontented and demoralized? Indeed, as it turns out in the novel, Marina's friend Danielle—the very one who could not imagine being in Marina's situation—is far from happy following a path of relentless "maturity" and independence. Working through this kind of narrative reauthoring, Marina could use psychotherapy to rework the meaning of the childhood metaphor, to develop new plot structures for her life, and to reconsider her narrative identifications. Narrative psychotherapy would accordingly allow her to reach a new level of peace with her current life and a new degree of flexibility as she makes plans for the future.

NARRATIVE PSYCHOTHERAPY INTEGRATION

The second way that narrative theory can be helpful for psychotherapy (and the one that is most important for narrative psychiatry) is to provide a metanarrative frame for psychotherapy integration (Angus and McLeod 2004; Hoshmand 2000; Richert 2006). I have touched on this aspect of narrative theory in the discussion of the history of psychotherapy and the recent move toward psychotherapeutic integration and eclecticism. Narrative psychotherapy integration helps make sense of the diversity of psychotherapies and provides a conceptual handle on many of the common factors within them. In this way, narrative theory provides an ideal tool for conceptualizing the insights of the Dodo bird verdict, evidence-based therapy, and postmodern theoretical work.

The basic idea behind a metanarrative integration is that all therapies, regardless of their specific orientation, contain what narrative psychologist Michele Crossely calls a "therapeutic narrative" (Crossely 2000, 163). All therapies start by listening to the stories clients tell and then using "therapeutic narratives" to help clients gain a new perspective on their situation and new tools for coping with their problems. Each of the many different therapeutic approaches, though they may be remarkably different in their particulars, use the structural elements of narrative (metaphor, plot, character, and point of view) to help people reauthor their stories. This will be as true in psychoanalysis as it is in cognitive behavioral, interpersonal, family, feminist, or even narrative psychotherapy. From the perspective of narrative psychotherapy integration, which approach to choose, or which combination of approaches, will depend on the goals of the client. There is no single or necessary approach to take. Many differing possibilities will yield many different lived realities. Which one to choose depends on the client's goals and desires.

This availability of many different approaches to psychotherapy means that when people enter psychotherapy they enter a critical moment of choice and self-determination. They enter a moment when politics and ethics are at the heart of their decision making. Empirical data and scientific research are relevant but not determinative. Much more critical for deciding is the wisdom of human meaning making and inescapability of human particularity one learns from literature, philosophy, and cultural study. Because narrative psychotherapy integration has a deep appreciation of this point, its relation to science is closer to the worldview of humanistic psychotherapy than to that of, say, cognitive behavioral therapy.

I should be clear, however, that not all approaches to psychotherapy integration share this humanistic preference. Some integrative therapists prefer to put their faith in science for navigating psychotherapeutic diversity. Norcross and Beutler, for example, argue that without relying on science integrative therapists risk falling into what they call "syncretism"— haphazard, uncritical, untrained, and unsystematic approaches to therapy (Norcross and Beutler 2008, 483). To avoid this fate, these therapists turn to "empirical knowledge and scientific research" to ground their integrative efforts (2008, 484). But privileging science is not the only way to avoid the risks of "syncretism." Another way is to develop a deeper understanding of the meaning of psychotherapeutic diversity through human study. Narrative theorists agree that the risk of doing therapy badly may be real, but this risk does not mean that science alone will save the day.

In this way, narrative psychotherapy integration echoes recent work sociologists have done on the critical role of politics and ethics in self-identification. Sociologist Anthony Giddens describes "life politics" as a politics of self-fashioning in the context of multiculturalism (Giddens 1991). The global multicultural diffusion of fixed tradition and hierarchical domination means that people must be increasingly self-reflexive in their self-determination and their lifestyle choices. Self-fashioning in this context becomes a political process, a politics of choice and a politics of life decisions. And, as we saw in the last chapter, sociologist Arthur Frank found that this is true not only with regard to the self narratives about career, family, religion, politics, and so on but also with regard to how people understand their illnesses. Illness, particularly chronic illness, can become a central aspect of a life story. When this happens, people must devote extensive resources of self-narration to understand what the illness means for their life. For Frank, the telling of an "illness narrative" is a deeply ethical moment that involves a perpetual self-monitoring and "a profound assumption of personal responsibility" (Frank 1995).

It is important to add that even though narrative psychotherapy integration does not put science first, this does not imply anything-goes relativism or that any old therapeutic interpretation will do. Narrative psychotherapy integration does not mean that the therapist can say things completely out of context like "Your problem is because the cow jumped over the moon." Rather, for psychotherapy to be effective, the therapist and the client must have a sense of belief and confidence in their interpretive frames.

To understand this nonrelativist aspect of narrative integration, it helps to recall the importance of two of Lambert's nonspecific therapeutic factors: common therapeutic features and client expectations. Psychotherapy researchers have developed their understanding of these nonspecific factors by focusing on the related concept of "therapeutic alliance." The concept of therapeutic alliance combines "both the therapist and the client contributions and emphasizes the partnership between client and therapist to achieve the clients goals" (Duncan 2002a, 39).[7] The critical importance of therapeutic alliance means that therapists do not have free range of options and they cannot just say or do anything. Therapists can maintain an alliance and foster a partnership only if they help develop interpretations that make sense to the client and that are consistent with the client's goals and expectations (Duncan and Miller 2000).

The real world matters in developing these interpretations, but the real world is complex enough that it allows considerable flexibility with regard to which aspect to focus on. From the perspective of narrative theory, different interpretations provide different metaphorical truths: different structures of understanding, different focuses of worldly attention, and different values, attitudes, and behaviors consistent with the different priorities of the interpretation selected. All of these factors mean that therapists do not have free play of interpretation. Their interventions are constrained by the real world, by the client's worldviews, and by the client's willingness to consider novel possibilities in the context of a therapeutic alliance. And yet even though there is not a free play of meaning, these constraints still allow considerable flexibility about which interpretation, or a combination of interpretations, will be useful and desirable.

These insights into narrative flexibility and narrative constraints fit well with Dodo bird outcome study research. This research opens easily to an understanding of therapy as a process in which client and therapist work together in the co-construction of meaning. As Hubble and colleagues put it in their summary of the Dodo bird insights for the therapeutic alliance, psychotherapy should be seen as a "partnership for change. It is a process that the client and therapist do together, rather than something done to the client. . . . In a well-functioning alliance, therapists and clients jointly work to construct interventions that are in accordance with client's preferred outcomes" (Hubble, Duncan, and Miller 1999, 416).

Conclusion

If we apply these insights to Marina's situation, we can see that narrative psychotherapy integration is tremendously useful for helping Marina consider the question of which psychotherapy to choose. Narrative integration can help Marina see that her choice between alternative psychotherapies is less about knowing which is superior across time and space and more about which therapy or combination of therapies fits best with her goals and desires. Marina's choice of therapeutic options is momentous because the kind of therapy she engages will be a major factor in shaping the kinds of problems she addresses and the kinds of solutions that are offered. Despite the importance of this choice, most psychotherapies spend little time considering the issues at stake. They dive into the details without thinking through the options. In contrast, narrative integration of psychotherapy brings the question of choice into the therapeutic process itself. A narrative integration of psychotherapy starts, in other words, with a consideration of where to start.

As one might imagine, there are many practical issues surrounding the use of narrative theory for psychotherapy integration. We will work through these issues in the later chapters where we look in further detail at a specific case example. But before turning to these clinical specifics, we must first work through the relevance of a narrative turn for psychiatry itself. As we will see, narrative psychiatry combines insights from narrative medicine and narrative psychotherapy integration. In addition, narrative psychiatry works through the issue of psychotropic drugs in a way that goes beyond medicine or psychotherapy. The medication question in narrative psychiatry means that questions of choice, therapeutic option, and life politics become even more complicated in narrative psychiatry.

CHAPTER FOUR

Narrative Psychiatry

H AVING REVIEWED THE EMERGENCE of narrative medicine and narrative approaches to psychotherapy integration, we are now in a position to draw out the implications for narrative psychiatry. The history of psychiatry has led to its own conceptual knots and practical predicaments. As for narrative medicine and narrative psychotherapy integration, the turn to narrative provides a way out of these difficulties. This chapter starts with a story of psychiatry's beginnings leading to its current conundrums. It follows with a discussion of the similarities and differences between narrative medicine, narrative psychotherapy integration, and narrative psychiatry.

A Brief Story of Psychiatry

My story of modern psychiatry does not begin with Flexner or Freud. Instead, it begins in late nineteenth-century Germany with Emil Kraepelin and what many call the first era of "biological psychiatry" (Shorter 1997, 69). Researchers in this era argued that "mental illnesses are brain diseases," and they advocated a clinical-pathological research method that extrapolated back and forth between clinical findings and autopsy findings (Fulford, Thornton, and Graham 2006, 152; Porter 2002, 144; Shorter 1997, 73–76). Emil Kraepelin brought this method to international attention when he used it to set up a psychiatric department in Munich that contemporary psychiatrists Nancy Andreasen and Donald Black call "one of the greatest departments of psychiatry of all time" (Andreasen and Black 1995, 9). The department included such neurological and psychiatric luminaries as Alois Alzheimer, Franz Nissl, and Korbinian Brodmann, and in the early decades of the twentieth century, their work was the nodal point for a period of tremendous optimism in psychiatric research.

These researchers firmly believed that systematic use of the clinical-pathological method would discover brain abnormalities that lay behind major psychiatric conditions. Kraepelin fueled this optimism by his success articulating a clinical distinction between dementia praecox (later called schizophrenia) and manic depressive illness which is still used to this day. And, even more, the optimism was fueled by the neuropathological discovery of two organic mental disorders: Alzheimer disease and general paralysis (syphilis of the brain). These last two discoveries were "world changing" events—"for the first time a specific psychiatric disease had been shown to have a specific neuropathological cause"—and the race was on to replicate similar findings throughout psychiatry (Fulford, Thornton, and Graham 2006, 152).

Despite this optimism, further research yielded little in the way of useful findings. Biological psychiatrists pressed on, undaunted by their limited findings, and continued to push their neurobiologic models. They pushed so hard and the models eventually became so fantastic that their colleagues started condescendingly referring to them as "Brain Mytholo gies" (Fulford, Thornton, and Graham 2006, 153). By the late 1920s, alternative approaches gained increasing attention, and the first era of biological psychiatry lost its pride of place.

The two most important alternatives were Sigmund Freud's psychoanalysis and Karl Jaspers's phenomenological psychiatry. Of the two, Freud's psychoanalysis was the most popular and also most radical break from biological psychiatry. Even though Freud started out as a neurologist and early on had also hoped that brain science would explain psychiatric problems, he eventually had to abandon this goal. A major factor in Freud's abandonment of brain research was fiscal necessity. Because Freud was forced into clinical practice to make a living (rather than academic research) and because patients with psychoneurotic complaints were the most available, Freud developed a clinical practice specializing in psychoneurosis. This meant that he had to quickly develop methods of treatment for these patients. As Freud put it, "Anyone who wants to make a living from the treatment of nervous patients must clearly be able to do something to help them" (Freud 1959, 16). The only treatments available at the time were electrotherapy and hypnotism. Freud found electrotherapy to be completely unhelpful, so he turned to hypnotherapy and eventually to "psycho-analysis" (1959, 30).

Freud's turn to hypnotherapy and psychoanalysis was a historic choice because it meant that he had to "abandon the treatment of organic nervous diseases" (1959, 17). Leaving behind his earlier work in neurology, Freud turned instead to understanding his patients' experiences. He put the same painstaking attention into understanding the interpretive links of his patient's psychic life as the biological psychiatrists had put into cataloging symptoms and examining brains. He did not, however, take the next step and consider the philosophical issues at stake in such a move. Whether because of his temperament or owing to the contingencies of his practice, Freud had little patience for the methodological or philosophical complications of this turn from organic to psychic analysis. He titled his first major book the *Interpretation of Dreams* (1900), but he had no background in the theory and method of interpretation and even less interest in gaining this expertise. He ignored the interpretive theories and methods from other disciplines (such as philosophy, history, and hermeneutics), and he "harshly denounced methodologists as people who spend all of their time cleaning their eyeglasses without ever looking through them" (Rubovits-Seitz 1998, 18). Freud was determined not to make this mistake.

Karl Jaspers's phenomenological psychiatry can be considered Freud's mirror image in this regard. Jaspers's contribution began in 1908 when he joined the then biologically minded psychiatry department in Heidelberg. Jaspers shared with biological psychiatrists of the time a general enthusiasm for empirical research, but he also considered biological research one-sided and believed that the obsession with brain research had gone too far. Jaspers's response to this situation differed considerably from Freud's. Instead of diving into meaning-centered analysis without pausing for philosophical or methodological reflection, Jaspers had the temperament and academic support to pull back from the particulars of patient care and consider the larger philosophical and methodological questions at issue. The most important question for Jaspers was the most basic: because psychiatry is primarily about humans, *what is the best way to study humans?* The next most important question followed directly from this: should inquiries about humans follow the methods of natural science (like the biological psychiatrists of his time), or is there something unique about humans that requires unique forms of inquiry (different from those found in natural sciences)?

To answer these questions, Jaspers turned to the leading thinkers of his time in the area of human inquiry—particularly Edmund Husserl (founder of philosophical phenomenology), Max Weber (a founder of sociology), and William Dilthey (a leading figure in cultural history and hermeneutics). Jaspers never adopted the views of these thinkers in total, but he did agree with their basic premise—that natural science methods alone were insufficient for human studies. Human inquiry, including psychiatric inquiry, was different from natural inquiry because it involved more than a study of cause and effect. It also involved a thick and subtle study of human systems of meaning. In short, to understand humans, one must not only *explain* their physical properties and causal laws but also *understand* their lived experience and their meaning systems—a task that the natural sciences did not have to contend with in the same way (Jaspers 1997; Phillips 2004).

Jaspers argued for a pluralistic version of psychiatry—a psychiatry that tended to both physical explanations and human understandings. He was critical of Freud's psychoanalysis because he felt that Freud lumped together explanation and understanding in an undifferentiated mix. For Jaspers, Freud seemed to have little appreciation that he was developing a meaning-centered psychiatry that required a particular approach that in no way excluded other approaches. Jaspers, in contrast, argued for both causal research (such as neuroanatomical or genetic causation) and meaning research (such as the type carried out in psychoanalysis). In addition, Jaspers argued for a psychiatry that remained open to philosophy and broader intellectual thought instead of becoming narrowly specialized in clinical or neuroscience literature alone. For these reasons, Jaspers has had a revival in contemporary philosophical psychiatry.

At the time he was working in psychiatry, however, Jaspers had only limited success. His monumental 1913 textbook *General Psychopathology* (Jaspers 1997) was well received, but the field as a whole had little patience for his theoretical endeavors. The temperament of psychiatry was much more similar to Freud's in this regard. Jaspers's work was considered overintellectual and therefore uninteresting. As one of his colleagues put it, "Too bad about Jaspers, such an intelligent fellow and engages in such monkey business" (quoted in Jaspers 1981, 22). Jaspers soon left psychiatry altogether to focus on philosophy.

While Jaspers's phenomenological psychiatry languished, Freud's psychoanalysis flourished. The growth of psychoanalysis had partly to do with Freud's pragmatic focus on treatment issues (as compared with Jaspers), but it also had to do with the tremendous influence Freud had looking through his interpretive eyeglasses (even if they were a little "dirty" by Jaspers's standards). Freud quickly developed a series of compelling insights into human psychic life that were hard to ignore. Concepts such as repression, resistance, mental conflict, ambivalence, unconscious, conversion, free association, infantile sexuality, libido, transference, dream work, manifest verses latent dream content, the Oedipal complex, narcissism, and ego, id, and superego became the lingua franca of not only psychiatry but also the era. Riding on these fruitful ideas and the excitement they generated, psychoanalysis eventually reached the height of its success in the 1960s (Zaretsky 2005, 11). By this time, most practicing psychiatrists in the United States considered themselves psychoanalytically oriented. Although only 10 percent had formal psychoanalytic training, those 10 percent were in positions of tremendous influence. They held virtually all the psychiatric departmental chairs, were key contributors to psychiatric education, and wrote many of the textbooks of the time.

This psychoanalytic prominence was short lived, however, and by 1980 the tide had turned dramatically back toward biopsychiatry.[1] The year 1980 marks the watershed for several reasons. The most obvious is that was the year the American Psychiatric Association published the third edition of its *Diagnostic and Statistical Manual of Mental Disorders* (*DSM-III*). At the time, Nancy Andreasen hailed *DSM-III* as a revolutionary book that would lead "to a massive reorganization and modernization of psychiatric diagnosis" (Andreasen 1984, 155). True to her prediction, historian of psychiatry Edwin Shorter echoed the same themes years later when he argued that *DSM-III* signaled a "turning of the page on psychoanalysis" and "a redirection of the discipline toward a scientific course" (Shorter 1997, 302).

The leading explanation for this switch is the "progress" of science, but as I discussed in the Preface, the impetus for the shift from psychoanalysis to biopsychiatry went far beyond science. Additional factors included the rise of psychopharmacologic treatments (such as Thorazine and imipramine), the corresponding creation of "chemical imbalance" theories of mental illness (such as the dopamine hypothesis for schizophrenia and the amine hypothesis for depression), increasing pressure from insurance companies to limit payments to operationally defined conditions, reaction from the psychiatric leadership to a host of "antipsychiatry" critiques, and an argumentative attack on psychoanalysis from philosophers of science who claimed that psychoanalysis had little more value than astrology.

I entered psychiatric training during the process of this paradigm switch, so I was able to watch it happen from the trenches. To me it seemed that even more important than the factors just mentioned was the extremely tight link between the interests of biological psychiatry and those of the rising pharmaceutical industry. The year 1980 provides a useful marker once again. Marcia Angell, the former editor and chief of the *New England Journal of Medicine*, explains that before 1980 the pharmaceutical industry "was a good business, but afterward it was a stupendous one" (Angell 2005, 3). Drug sales were fairly steady from 1960 to 1980, but during the next twenty years sales tripled to more than $200 billion a year (2005, 3). The year 1980 is the watershed for the pharmaceutical industry because in one sweep it brought the election of Ronald Reagan, a new business-friendly climate in Congress, and the passage of several probusiness legislations (such as the Bayh-Dole Act, designed to speed technology transfers from tax-supported universities to the corporations). In the wake of these changes, the pharmaceutical industry unleashed a marketing blitz of staggering proportions that has only grown in recent years.

The most well-known tools of this marketing blitz are *direct-to-consumer* (DTC) and *direct-to-provider* (DTP) advertising that now saturate the lay and professional media. The less well-known tools of the marketing blitz are *indirect-to-consumer* (ITC) and *indirect-to-provider* (ITP) promotions. These indirect methods follow the basic public relations tactic known as the "third man" technique—where promotion comes indirectly through a seemingly neutral "third man" and therefore sidesteps the usual scrutiny and skepticism people give to direct advertising (Rampton and Stauber 2002). For consumers, indirect promotional practices include press and video news releases, product placement techniques, and the setting up of various patient and disease-specific advocacy groups (which allow products to be promoted without it seeming like the promotion comes from the corporations directly). For providers, they include an avalanche of promotion in the form of continuing medical education materials, medical opinion leaders, and medical practice and treatment guidelines. Indeed, even the science of medicine itself has in many ways become a marketing arm of the pharmaceutical companies (Smith 2005).

This transition of the pharmaceutical industry into a corporate colossus right at the same time that psychiatry moved into its second biological era is not a coincidence. The rise of the pharmaceuticals had a huge impact not only on psychiatry but also on the whole of medical education and research. As Angell explains, they effectively transformed the "ethos of medical schools and teaching hospitals. These nonprofit institutions started to see themselves as 'partners' of industry and they became just as enthusiastic as any entrepreneur about the opportunities to parlay their discoveries into financial gain" (Angell 2005, 8). All of medicine was targeted, but psychiatry in particular provided an ideal site for manipulation. The vast bulk of the increased sales after 1980 were those of lifestyle drugs and me-too drugs devoted to chronic conditions, and that meant psychiatry was the perfect focus. Psychiatry, in other words, provided pharmaceutical public relations experts with a corporate "marketer's dream" (2005, 88).

Whether psychiatry would have moved into a repetition of its first biological era without the pharmaceuticals is an unknown question. But certainly the money and influence of the pharmaceuticals put a heavy thumb on the scale of history, and by the year 2000 psychiatry was fully in the grips of a second biological era. Once again, psychiatric leadership changed, and biological psychiatrists regained all the key positions. And, once again, the narrow-mindedness of this approach created a host of critiques and unrest. Contemporary critiques of the second era of biopsychiatry are now coming from both outside and within the profession. Outside the profession, these include renewed consumer/survivor grassroots activism and the mobilization of a range of cultural studies critiques coming from academics in the humanities and social sciences. Within the profession, they have taken the form of a revival of Jaspers-style philosophy and psychiatry, the emergence of "postpsychiatry" critiques that stand on the shoulders of contemporary social theory, and the development of a critical psychiatry network (mostly in the United Kingdom but rapidly spreading around the globe). In addition, many of the critics of the second era of biopsychiatry have begun to coalesce and develop political clout around the rallying cry of "recovery in psychiatry." The recovery movement is working hard to reorient the field toward a more peer-based, person-centered, and holistic focus.[2]

As with the first era of biological psychiatry, many of the contemporary critiques involve a reaction against the increasing narrow-mindedness of psychiatric practice that comes from reducing human psychological life to primarily biological variables. In addition, the critiques involve a deep resistance to psychiatry's relentless disease mongering, its overuse of polypharmacy (relying, if necessary, on involuntary court mandates to enforce compliance), and its knee-jerk medicating for relatively minor difficulties not only in adults but also in children and adolescents—all of which are seen by contemporary critics as the result of biopsychiatry being effectively hijacked by pharmaceutical corporate interests.

The Emergence of Narrative Psychiatry

Understanding this history of psychiatry helps us appreciate the critical importance of narrative approaches. Narrative psychiatry enters the discourse of psychiatry at the same moment as these other critiques of biopsychiatry. But narrative psychiatry is less of a critique and more of a way forward in psychiatry. It provides a way for savvy educators, reformers, and practitioners to negotiate the contradictions in the field without falling into swirling polemics or developing rigid "anti-this" or "pro-that" dichotomies—such as antipsychiatry versus propsychiatry, or drug therapy versus talk therapy. The turn to narrative in psychiatry, in other words, serves to heal the current tensions in psychiatry not unlike the way the turn to narrative functions in both medicine and psychotherapy. For that reason, perhaps the best way to understand narrative psychiatry is to compare it with its sibling fields in medicine and psychotherapy that we reviewed in the last two chapters.

SIMILARITIES TO NARRATIVE MEDICINE AND NARRATIVE PSYCHOTHERAPY

Like narrative medicine, narrative psychiatry is a deeply person-centered practice that puts first and foremost the human importance of clinical stories. Psychiatric patients, like medical patients, are much more than a collection of biological variables. They come to the clinics with intensely personal stories to tell. The most important task of the narrative medicine, and therefore narrative psychiatry, is to be a good listener and to empathically connect with the person's story. Narrative psychiatrists, like narrative physicians, seek to understand the person they are working with as their primary objective. This narrative understanding brings patient and clinician together into a shared experience of the patient's world. It provides much more than a causal explanation of problem A or problem B, and it does not simply abstract from the person's situation a diagnostic label that would group all problems under a well-known abstract grid. Instead, narrative understanding tunes into the uniqueness of the individual and the unrepeatability of the person's experience and difficulties. Narrative understanding is a deep appreciation of the person as a whole, what it feels like for this person, in this particular context, going through these particular problems.

Psychiatrist Robert Coles captured this deeply person-centered dimension of psychiatric work in his book *The Mind's Fate: A Psychiatrist Looks at His Profession*. Coles, acclaimed as both physician and author (and in that way similar to Chekhov and Verghese), developed "a way of seeing psychiatry" over the course of his career that comes close to narrative psychiatry. Coles never worked out a narrative theory of psychiatry, but his work anticipates much of narrative psychiatry and provides a beacon for what psychiatry could look like if it tended more closely to the narrative, or "storied" (as Coles would have it), dimensions of psychic life and suffering.[3]

Coles argues that the person-centered core of narrative psychiatry is the "*ultimate mission* of those who are doctors of the mind." To be a psychiatrist, in other words, is to be an "attentive listener first." It is to have learned how to make sense of the "inside cry for a knowing assistance that is at the heart of a person's decision to visit a physician" (Coles 1995, xx; italics added). This kind of attentive listening remains central to psychiatry despite a century of insights into mind and brain because inescapably

> we human beings are creatures of awareness, of language, of long and articulated memory—and also, creatures whose special skills and triumphs live side by side with a special capacity for tragedy. Our losses, our vulnerabilities, our weak spots and soft spots, our ultimate

destiny of disappearance from this planet are known to us, as they are not to all other forms of life on this earth. Through words, whether spoken to others or silently put to ourselves, we constantly struggle to make sense of things, even as we try (if we can) to prepare ourselves for the worst: hunker or huddle down, reach out, whistle in the dark, while trembling mightily within ourselves. Not rarely, at such moments, we have learned in this century to seek the counsel of psychiatrists, men and women presumed to understand our many possible predicaments, our wild or loony sides, our lapses into incoherence or rage, into lusts and times of darkness that threaten our reliability, our stability, our very lives (or those of others). (Coles 1995, xx)

For Coles, psychiatrists must understand that to be sought out at these moments, to be asked to "attend such a cry" is an honor, a privilege, and the "ultimate bedrock" of psychiatry's professional competence (1995, xx).

By tuning in to the person's story, first and foremost, as a goal in and of itself, narrative psychiatrists, like their narrative medicine colleagues, create an environment in which the person can be known and his or her difficulties appreciated. This step alone can be one of the most healing acts a clinician can perform. When clinicians allow the person to be known in this way, they form a bond that reduces the patient's isolation because the patient immediately becomes less alone with his or her problem. Whatever else may happen in the clinical encounter, this sense of togetherness will reduce the person's suffering. The patient now has a comrade, a foxhole partner, someone who is in it with him or her. This partnership may not change the extent of the person's troubles, but it changes immensely the experience of the situation.

Although clinicians are not the only ones who can perform this role, a good clinician can sometimes be one of the few people in the person's world who can truly understand. Clinicians have extensive background with similar experiences of human suffering, as well as the advantage of working in clinical settings where many of the barriers to discussing shameful or embarrassing problems often come down.

Going further and following the lead of narrative psychotherapy integration, narrative psychiatrists also tune in to the way that the stories people tell about themselves not only describe their lives but also shape their lives. The stories people use to frame and organize their life situation are not simply incidental to their identity; they are the primary tools people have for configuring their identity. Narrative psychiatry, like narrative psychotherapy integration, recognizes that the shaping of identity through narrative is a major tool for recovery. When people come for help in a therapeutic situation, they not only want to be understood but also often want help to make changes in their lives. Narrative psychiatry, like narrative psychotherapy integration, understands that reworking the stories people tell about themselves is a powerful way to make changes and to reauthor their lives.

The narrative turn in psychiatry therefore works like the narrative turn in psychotherapy integration in that it provides a metatheoretical frame that allows psychiatrists to appreciate a range of different psychotherapy approaches. Narrative psychiatry, like narrative psychotherapy integration, appreciates that the many competing forms of psychotherapy are alternative ways to tell the story of psychic life and psychic suffering. Navigating this diversity is less about trying to figure out which form of psychotherapy is "true" and "best" for all people and more about understanding which is "truest" and most "valuable" for the person who is using therapy to organize his or her life. In short, the question is not whether any one of these diverse options or some combination of them is ultimately correct. The question is how they might have a role in working with a particular person.

DIFFERENCES FROM NARRATIVE MEDICINE AND NARRATIVE PSYCHOTHERAPY INTEGRATION

Although there are similarities between narrative medicine, narrative psychotherapy integration, and narrative psychiatry, there are important differences as well. The major difference between these fields comes from the more prominent consideration of psychiatric medications in narrative psychiatry than in the other two domains. The use of psychiatric medications is symbolic of a much larger philosophical issue having to do with the way these different fields approach the "disease" versus "illness" distinction. The disease/illness distinction, which is related to Karl Jaspers's distinction between *explanation* and *understanding*, differentiates the explanations of medicine and science (disease) from the understandings of human experience and suffering (illness). The distinction has long roots in Western culture going back to at least the time of Cartesian dualism between body and mind, and it is at the heart of important differences between the practices of narrative medicine, narrative psychotherapy integration, and narrative psychiatry.

Narrative medicine and narrative psychotherapy integration tend to sidestep the issue and function with the disease/illness distinction largely intact. Narrative psychiatry, in contrast, must be able to negotiate the distinction directly and with subtlety.[4] Narrative psychiatry cannot sidestep the disease/illness distinction because of the psychiatric medication question and also because the distinction, as Jaspers argued one hundred years ago, sits at the heart of psychiatry. In psychiatry, people's suffering, their illness experience, often becomes their "disease," and the two concepts are deeply intertwined. Indeed, the whole conceptual intermingling of the terms "mental disease" and "mental illness" rests on a blurred distinction between disease and illness. The phrase "depression is a disease"—which has become the ubiquitous slogan of antistigma campaigns—captures this situation perfectly. The illness experience of depression is the disease that psychiatry addresses.

But just because mainstream psychiatry sits at the heart of the disease/illness distinction does not mean it has developed the sophisticated conceptual tools needed to deal with the distinction. Indeed, psychiatrists in general, like their colleagues in medicine and psychotherapy, tend to keep the distinction pretty much intact and have great difficulty thinking outside this binary. The main difference is that it works less well in psychiatry and leaves psychiatrists in a more uncomfortable conceptual zone. Or worse, as Jaspers argued, psychiatry's clumsiness with this distinction all too often leaves psychiatrists caught up in an "intellectual jumble" and a "chaotic diversity of viewpoints" that for Jaspers meant only one thing: "Psychiatrists must learn to think" (Jaspers 1981, 208). Narrative psychiatry takes up Jaspers's charge and works to bring much more nuance and self-reflection to the disease/illness distinction.

Narrative theory provides several important tools for navigating the complications of the disease/illness distinction. Starting with the concepts of plot and emplotment, narrative theory provides key tools for negotiating the conundrum of the disease/illness distinction. One of the most remarkable aspects of plot, as we discussed in the last chapter, is that it can bring together into a single story vastly different kinds of logics and phenomena. Thus, it is not uncommon to hear a story that brings together the mechanical explanatory logics of science with the experiential understanding of human psychic life.

Consider the following fictional story about Susan's desire to get back together with Ilene:

> *Susan wants more than anything else to reunite with Ilene. Ilene is skeptical; she still loves Susan but feels that Susan is too irresponsible for a committed relationship. After much pleading, Ilene finally agrees to give Susan one more chance and they plan a reconciliation meeting. Susan gets so excited that she forgets to put gas in her car and ends up stranded on the side of the road with no way to make the meeting. Ilene goes home exasperated vowing never to have romantic connections with Susan again.*

This story combines an array of seemingly disconnected phenomena regarding Susan: her desire for reunion, her character traits, her forgetfulness, the complexities of her relationship with Ilene, and the mechanical failure of her car. Yet we have no trouble understanding the story or how all these fit together in Susan's situation. The same is true for the disease/illness distinction. If we added to this story information about Susan's biology or her neurobiology and how that is affecting her life with Ilene, we could still understand it. Suppose, for example, Susan forgot to take her seizure medication in all the excitement and had a seizure the day of her meeting with Ilene. We could easily plot this neurobiologic information alongside the other information. Plotted stories, in other words, have no trouble combining human experience, human desires, and human character traits with medical explanatory logics of science and disease.

In addition to plot, narrative brings considerable nuance to the disease/illness distinction through its appreciation of the role of metaphor and linguistic structure for human meaning. Whether we are talking about disease or illness, the common ground between the two is that they are both forms of meaning making. Disease makes meaning one way, illness another way. But they are both meanings, and they both rely on the tools of language to shape their meaning. Although this concept might be readily acceptable with regard to illness, many would object to it with regard to disease. Metaphor and linguistic structure may shape ordinary human meanings, many would argue, but science is exceptional. A forceful state-ment of this type with regard to disease and illness comes from Susan Sontag in her book *Illness as Metaphor* (Sontag 1978). For Sontag, people experience illness in terms of metaphor, but disease itself is not metaphor—disease is the truth. She argues that metaphor leads to all kinds of mis-understandings and confusions because, for Sontag, the most truthful way to be ill is to cleanse oneself of all metaphorical thinking and to rely solely on the nonmetaphorical disease thinking of medicine and science.

But is disease thinking really free of metaphor, and is the meaning mak-ing of science really an exception to other forms of meaning making? Most science studies scholars would say no. Science, including medical science, is a particular kind of human meaning making, and metaphor provides one of the easiest ways to see the similarity of meaning making both within and outside science. Metaphor enters science at its core through science's inescapable use of models to organize its research. These scientific models work much the same way that metaphors work—they explain the world through a metaphorical redescription (Hesse 2000, 353). For example, just as the metaphor "man is a wolf" redescribes man in a new way and allows us to perceive something new about him, the medical model of mental ill-ness—"depression is a disease"—redescribes depression and allows us to perceive something new about it. The initial value of scientific models is quite like the surprise of a fresh metaphor. The difference between a poetic metaphor and a scientific model, however, is that scientific models are more patiently pursued, used to inform an entire work or movement, whereas the poet uses the metaphor for only a quick glimpse (Burke 1954, 96).

Finally, narrative helps provide nuance to the disease/illness distinction through the concept of narrative identity. Narrative identity recognizes the tremendous variability of human identifications and joins with a li-brary of contemporary scholarship that troubles the notion of human identity as fixed or essential. From a narrative perspective, we form our identifications through the stories we tell about ourselves, and those sto-ries are shaped and organized by the plots and metaphors we use. It fol-lows that narrative identifications can use plots containing disease logics and disease metaphors as easily as they can use other logics and meta-phors. Thus the concept of narrative identity gives us insight into how we can learn to tell self stories and create self-understandings out of the logics of science and medicine. There is nothing theoretically exceptional about science and medicine here. Science and medicine can be brought into narrative identifications as well as any other story elements.

That said, however, something culturally exceptional is going on with today's neurobiologic forms of self-making. Medical models of mind are becoming so rapidly prominent in our culture that social theorist have started to coin new terms to describe them. Anthropologist Emily Martin uses the phrase "pharmaceutical person" and sociologist Nicholas Rose uses the term "neurochemical self" to describe this emerging form of neuro-chemically mediated identity (Martin 2006; Rose 2003). To become a neurochemical self, these cultural scholars argue, one does not have to become a fundamentally different kind of human. One only has to internalize the logics of neuroscience and the practices of psychopharmacology and use these logics and practices to organize one's sense of self.

Consider this example from Jonathan Franzen's novel *The Corrections*:

Although in general Gary applauded the modern trend toward individual self-management of retirement funds and long-distance calling plans and private-schooling options, he was less than thrilled to be given responsibility for his own personal brain chemistry, especially when certain people in his life, notably his father, refused to take any such responsibility. But Gary was nothing if not conscientious. As he entered the darkroom, he estimated that his levels of Neurofactor 3 (i.e., serotonin: a very, very important factor) were posting seven-day or even thirty-day highs, that his Factor 2 and Factor 7 levels were likewise outperforming expectation, and that his Factor 1 had rebounded from an early-morning slump related to the glass of Armagnac he'd drunk at bedtime. He had a spring in his step, and agreeable awareness of his above-average height and his late summer suntan. His resentment of his wife, Caroline, was moderate and well contained. Declines led key advances in key indices of paranoia (e.g., his persistent suspicion that Caroline and his two older sons were mocking him), and his seasonally adjusted assessment of life's futility and brevity was consistent with the overall robustness of his mental economy. He was not the least clinically depressed. (Franzen 2001, 139–40)

Whatever else we might want to say about Gary, it's clear that the metaphors and plots of neuroscience have become a core part of his self-understanding.

For another example, this time from "real life" rather than fiction, consider this quotation from neurophilosopher Patricia Churchland as she describes her feelings to Paul (her neurophilosopher husband) after a particularly hard day at the university: "Pat burst in the door, having come straight from a frustrating faculty meeting. She said, 'Paul, don't speak to me, my serotonin levels have hit bottom, my brain is awash in glucocorticoids, my blood vessels are full of adrenaline, and if it weren't for my endogenous opiates I'd have driven the car into a tree on the way home. My dopamine levels need lifting. Pour me a Chardonnay, and I'll be down in a minute'" (MacFarquhar 2007, 69). Neurochemical selves like these are selves like other selves. The main difference is that they are rapidly incorporating different metaphors, plots, and narrative identifications than are non-neurochemical selves.

All of this comes directly into play whenever psychiatric medications are used to treat mental conditions because a medication intervention goes hand in hand with a neurochemical self. Narrative psychiatrists do not denigrate this form of self-making as more mythic (and therefore somehow less true) than other forms of self-making, but narrative psychiatrists do have a nuanced relationship with rapidly expanding neurochemical selves. On the one hand, narrative psychiatrists are open to this form of self-making and respect it as much as they would other forms of self. On the other hand, they are also aware of the often problematic power dynamics of this emerging form of self. Both Nicolas Rose and Emily Martin point to contemporary pharmaceutical practices as a major determinant of this new form of self-making. And, as I discussed above, pharmaceuticals are notorious in their willingness to use public relations and marketing techniques—including a co-optation of psychiatric science and psychiatric treatment protocols—in their relentless pursuit of profits and market share. The pharmaceuticals, as a result, increasingly dominate other forms of self-making, and their message tends to drown out other options.

For narrative psychiatrists, the contemporary incitement to become a "pharmaceutical person" becomes grist for the mill, as psychoanalysts like to say, in the clinical setting. Narrative psychiatrists navigate their complicated relationship to pharmaceutical self-making by sharing with their clients their ambivalence during their discussion of drug treatment options. They let their clients know that there is considerable hype regarding psychiatric medications, and they make it a point to discuss the side effect risks and questionable efficacy of many these medications. However, they also make it clear that, for any one person, there is no way to know—except through a treatment trial—how much a particular person might benefit or risk from a medication. Should the patient wish to undertake such a trial in the context of informed decision making, the narrative psychiatrist is willing to provide whatever assistance he or she can. For narrative psychiatrists, psychopharmacologic frames and strategies are one of an array of possible tools that can be woven together into an eclectic narrative of treatment. The baggage of their largely corporate production and marketing does not necessarily rule out their usefulness for a particular person in a particular situation.

Clearly, however, the disease model of mental suffering is not the only model available for self-making in psychiatry. There are a number of others, such as psychoanalytic, existential, cognitive, social, and spiritual models. As we shall see, all these models will be important for narrative psychiatrists. Narrative psychiatrists are not surprised that the understanding of human situations may involve mechanical logics or that key metaphors (whether psychoanalytic or cognitive or family or even biological) can play a part in human identifications. Narrative psychiatry allows psychiatrists to be sufficiently flexible that they can move with comfort in and between these many logics and metaphors in their work. In this way, narrative psychiatry not only better negotiates the disease/illness binary but also moves past the long history of psychiatric factionalism and competing "orientations." Narrative psychiatry does not require psychiatrists to throw out their other skills and knowledge. It provides a flexible framework in which psychiatrists can understand the many logics in which they work.

Conclusion

Narrative psychiatry is an emergent form of psychiatry that tends to and heals many of the historical conundrums of contemporary psychiatry. It borrows from recent narrative turns at the cutting edge of both medicine and psychotherapy integration. Like narrative medicine, narrative psychiatry seeks a deep and empathic understanding of the patient as a person. Like narrative psychotherapy integration, it appreciates that the process of recovery often involves reauthoring and retelling the stories of our lives. Different from narrative medicine and psychotherapy, narrative psychiatry extends its narrative awareness to the use of psychiatric medications and includes a narrative appreciation of the disease/illness distinction. To do this, narrative psychiatrists are as self-reflexively adept at a narrative understanding of the many stories that psychiatrists tell as they are at understanding stories of psychic life that their clients tell. This understanding of the narrative dimension of psychiatric stories includes biopsychiatric stories of "chemical imbalances" and "genetic predisposition" as well as the many other options in the clinical literature (such as psychoanalysis, humanistic psychotherapy, and family therapy, just to name a few). It also includes the many options beyond the clinical literature (such as alternative healing practices as well as the many possibilities explored in fiction and memoir).

As a result, the turn to narrative in psychiatry provides a way forward that throws out much of the dogma and factionalism of contemporary psychiatry without discarding more than one hundred years of research and clinical inquiry. Furthermore, the turn to narrative in psychiatry opens psychiatry to range of additional resources in the academy. The knowledge base of narrative psychiatry includes not only the sciences and quantitative social sciences but also ethnography, philosophy, history, literature, the arts, and consumer perspectives. All these resources come together to enhance narrative psychiatrists' capacity to help people understand the stories of their lives and imagine restoried alternatives that provide not only a new sense of meaning but also new possibilities for future action.

CHAPTER FIVE

Mrs. Dutta and the Literary Case

N ARRATIVE PSYCHIATRY INSIGHTS become clearer when we use them to consider case examples. Through case examples, narrative theory becomes concrete and the relevance of narrative psychiatry is brought vividly to life. Case examples also demonstrate much of the wisdom of narrative theory because they tell a story about a person and that story is necessarily shaped by the tools of narrative I have discussed: plot, metaphor, character, and point of view. In addition, case examples provide an opportunity to imagine an array of ways in which a person's story could be framed or reframed.

Choosing case examples for teaching narrative psychiatry is no simple matter, however, because any case one would choose is already framed in a particular narrative form. This means that much of the "work" of narrative framing—which is at the heart of narrative psychiatry—has been done in advance. The ideal case for narrative psychiatry would remain as open as possible and allow for as many readings as possible. Case examples originating from the clinical literature rarely fit this ideal because they are too often framed in a way that feels heavy handed and that makes it difficult to imagine alternative frames. Consider, for example, the following clinical case from the *DSM-III Casebook*:

> A 50 year-old widow was transferred to a medical center from her community mental health center, to which she had been admitted three weeks previously with severe agitation, pacing, and hand wringing, depressed mood accompanied by severe self-reproach, insomnia, and a 6–8 kg (15-pound) weight loss. She believed that her neighbors were against her, had poisoned her coffee, and had bewitched her to punish her because of her wickedness. Seven years previously, after the death of her husband, she had required

hospitalization for a similar depression, with extreme guilt, agitation, insomnia, accusatory hallucinations of voices calling her a worthless person, and preoccupation with thoughts of suicide. (Spitzer, Skodol, Gibbon, and Williams 1981, 28)

This case example has been tightly organized to foreground *DSM-III* variables consistent with a diagnosis of "Major Depression with Psychotic Features." The story tells us that a woman has been transferred to a medical center from her community because of severe depression and that she went through something similar seven years earlier at the time of her husband's death. We learn almost nothing about the person in the story other than the presence of a checklist of *DSM-III* variables. All other aspects of the person and her situation have been abstracted away.

Borrowing a distinction from anthropologist Clifford Geertz, we can call these highly abstracted clinical stories "thin" stories (Geertz 1973, 7). Thin stories may be said to contrast with the "thick" stories of everyday life and the stories people first bring to a clinical encounter. In the example from the *DSM-III Casebook*, the story "the 50 year-old woman" first told her clinicians would no doubt be much thicker than the thin one presented in the *DSM-III*. The woman would have likely given a wealth of information about her troubles. Just listing the elements she might have discussed can seemingly go on forever. They might include her feelings about her neighbors, how they are out to get her, what started the tensions between them, what it is like to be a widow, her feelings about her husband and his death, what killed him at such an early age, what kind of grief she went through, what's going on with her family, children that she did or did not have, her attempts to date again and to find companionship and intimacy, how she spends her time during the days, what she cares about, what she watches on television, a commercial she saw for antidepressants, how she supports herself, the struggles she has had to finding meaningful work, the society that she lives in and how it supports her or does not, whether she has made an attempt to get involved in politics, the state of her apartment, her diet, her aches and pains, the economy, her financial situation, sexism, racism, how people at the community mental health center have treated her, how she ended up at the medical center, just to name a few.

One of the most important outcomes of standard, non-narrative clinical training is to create clinicians who are able to sort through a thick story like the one the "50 year-old widow" would tell and turn it into the kind of thin story that shows up in medical records and in the clinical literature. Indeed, there is a fascinating moment in Tanya Luhrmann's ethnography of psychiatric training when she describes the struggles that a young psychiatric resident goes through trying to abstract a thick patient narrative into a thin clinical story. Dr. Gertrude, as Luhrmann calls her, was a highly accomplished and competent medical intern, but when she came to the psychiatric wards for her first psychiatric admission, it took her four hours to do one write-up. Luhrmann describes her struggles this way:

> [Dr. Gertrude] had interviewed her first patient with a senior resident, and they had concluded that the patient had obsessive-compulsive disorder. She had the official diagnostic handbook for psychiatry, which she opened to the page on obsessive-compulsive disorder. She had a copy of another admission note for a patient with obsessive-compulsive disorder. She had a mass of notes on the patient she'd just interviewed. But after the patient had gone she stood behind the desk, her body tight and clenched, swaying slightly, desperate and terrified in her neat suit. (Luhrmann 2000, 31)

Dr. Gertrude was so awash in the thick details of the first story she heard that she found it nearly impossible to see how that story could be turned into the neat admission note example before her. Luhrmann describes this early training experience for Dr. Gertrude as nothing short of "panic." But Dr. Gertrude's panic was short lived. By the end of her first year in psychiatry, she was routinely doing a new interview and dictating an admission note in less than an hour. The whole thing became so natural and spontaneous that she found it hard to remember why it had been a problem in the first place.

Luhrmann argues that through pattern recognition, which she calls the "prototype effect," residents gradually learn to make diagnostic assessments almost instantly. Young psychiatrists learn to make a diagnosis with speed that is "more like recognizing chairs or tables than it is like pulling out a manual and carefully double-checking the printed criteria" (Luhrmann 2000, 42). After time, "doing a lot of diagnoses, using prototypes, and writing admission notes tends to give one the sense that there *are* underlying essences" to psychiatric diagnosis (2000, 44). The cumulative effect of the learning process implies that for each diagnosis there is an underlying disease, and before long "the inherent ambiguity of psychiatric diagnosis can rapidly disappear from the young psychiatrist's experience" (2000, 45).

The Literary Case

Because the stories clinicians tell and write tend to be of the thin variety (like Gertrude's or the one in the *DSM-III Casebook*), the clinical literature is usually not a good place to get initial case histories for narrative psychiatry exposition.[1] Once a clinician has sifted through a thick story and reduced it to a thin clinical tale, it can be extremely hard to imagine the story being told in any other way. The story the clinician tells comes to feel compelling, and the variables he or she has abstracted out come to seem irrelevant. For that reason, it is better to turn to fictional presentations for narrative psychiatry cases. Memoir and autobiography can be used as well, but these genres also tend to reduce ambiguity in the process of the telling of the narrative.

Even fictional presentations tell thin stories in the end, otherwise the fictional presentations would be just as long as the life they are describing (actually longer because each moment in a life could be described in thick detail that would last much longer than the moment itself). But even though fictional narratives are abstracted as well, relative to clinical tales, fictional authors, particularly literary fiction authors, tend to give their readers a much thicker set of contextual variables than one can find almost anywhere else outside the clinical encounter itself. It is for this reason that fictional narratives become the ideal place to gather case histories for developing narrative psychiatry insights and skills.

The use of fiction in psychiatry has a long history—going back at least to Freud's interpretations of Hamlet—and the use of literature in medical teaching has become a staple of work in medical humanities (Hawkins and McEntyre 2000; Jones 1991). For narrative psychiatry, I find that the most helpful strategy for using literature is the one developed by Columbia psychiatrist William Tucker (Tucker 1994). Tucker is not a narrative psychiatrist, but his method is adoptable for narrative purposes. He focuses his teaching on the short story because he finds that, compared with other literary genres, short stories are more accessible than poems and less time consuming than novels or plays. Tucker's goal for using fiction is to help the reader imagine doing clinical work with one of the characters in the story. He does not approach a story as a literary theorist but much as a clinician, and he asks the people he works with to begin their reflection on a story by selecting a central character on which to focus. He then asks the reader to try to understand the character's problems, how the problems evolve in the story, and what might be likely to happen in the character's future beyond the story. Finally, he asks the reader to imagine what might happen if the character came to work with an imaginary psychiatrist. In short, Tucker uses fiction to develop what we could call "literary case histories."

Unfortunately, Tucker's approach cannot be applied directly to narrative psychiatry because he asks his readers to frame the character's problems using Erik Erikson's life stages model. Tucker narrows his interpretive field to the work of Erikson because he finds his readers have considerable difficulty formulating the character's problems. "The possibilities are so varied," he laments, that they tend to overwhelm people (1994, 214). But for narrative psychiatry the variability of possible ways to understand a story is just the point. In teaching narrative psychiatry, rather than close down the options in advance by using Erikson's life stages model, or any other model, the idea is to keep the options as open as possible. This helps people develop an experiential understanding of the considerable degrees of freedom and agency they have with regard narrating life stories.

Nonetheless, Tucker's model is helpful, and I find a modified version extremely useful for teaching narrative psychiatry. Like Tucker, I start by asking readers to select a character on which to focus. Then I ask them to follow with the character the rising tensions the character experiences. This gives readers a sense of the character's problems in their temporal evolution rather than just in cross section. Literary fiction does not usually present characters as having static or stereotypical traits, but rather the characters are very much in process. The characters' experiences and the changes they go through are responses to a series of events and interactions described in the story. The value of adopting Tucker's method for narrative psychiatry is that it helps the reader see the multiplicity of interpretations that could be used to understand the character's development.

Bringing this multiplicity to life and helping readers imagine alternative ways to understand the character is the key goal of using stories for teaching narrative psychiatry.

In most short stories, the character's developmental arc follows the general plot outlines of Frietag's triangle: rising tension, crisis, resolution (Bell 1997, 29; Martin 1986). A story that follows this plot structure begins with a main character caught in a conflict that gets worse over the course of the story. The conflict then worsens to a point of crisis, a point where some change is forced on the character. Finally, in the resolution of the story, the character evolves and makes changes that resolve the previous tension and conflict.

When the story follows this plot structure, I ask readers to imagine that the character comes to see a psychiatrist during her time of crisis, before a resolution has been settled. Sometimes I find it helps to imagine with readers that the character's crisis has gotten worse than it did in the story. This way we get to discuss a narrative approach to severe crisis situations similar to the ones that psychiatrists often see. In earlier chapters, I used a similar method in my discussion of the character Danielle from Claire Messud's novel *The Emperor's Children*. Although novels do not work as well for teaching purposes (because they are too long for most students to complete in the time allotted), the characters often go through similar arcs. In the case of Danielle, she reached a crisis concerning her feelings of being "childish" that she resolved by getting married and getting a job. It is possible to imagine Danielle as a client who comes to see a clinician at the point of her crisis, and it is also possible to imagine that her crisis becomes much worse than it does in the fictional presentation itself.

If we take these imaginative steps, we are in an ideal situation to begin the further narrative work I call "developing future histories." A *future history* is a speculative history, a kind of fantasy projection, in which the clinician and client begin the process of imagining possible resolutions to the client's troubles. The work of developing future histories calls on both the clinician's and the client's most creative capacities because a future history involves a leap into the unknown, the possible rather than the actual. Although clinicians are familiar with obtaining "past histories," they are much less familiar with the idea of a future history, and they are generally given no instruction on how to develop their skills in this area. This is unfortunate because developing future histories—imagining viable outcomes for the client's situation—will be the most critical skill for helping clients discover and consider resolutions to their presenting troubles.

It is important to recognize that developing future histories is imaginative work rather than work of the will. In other words, the first task of clinicians and clients is to escape from the domination of the current story the client tells in order to imagine alternatives. Only after this imaginative work has been completed can alternative choices be made. As Paul Ricoeur puts it, "the power of allowing oneself to be struck by new possibilities precedes the power of making up one's mind and choosing" (Ricoeur 1991a, 101). Thus, the first step in a narrative psychiatry reading of fiction is the step of imagining new possibilities.

It is equally important to recognize that the new possibilities of narrative work are not developed out of nothing. They are developed in the crucible of cultural frames that are available to the client and the therapist. That means the therapist and client will need not only to explore the person's life but also to be curious about the world outside the client. They will need to be curious about the world of alternative possibilities for human troubles and to have a deep familiarity with these alternatives.

Where should narrative therapists turn to develop their familiarity with possible future histories? There are many places where these alternatives may be drawn. Certainly the stories that both the client and the therapist have heard over the course of their lifetime will be a rich source of narrative possibilities. In addition, the worlds of literature, theater, film, memoir, and biography all provide rich sources of narratives that might be useful. And, perhaps most important, the clinical literature itself—particularly if we define clinical literature broadly—can be an excellent source of narrative options. Although the clinical literature is not a good place to look for stories open to multiple interpretations, it is an excellent source for finding resources for narrative meaning. The clinical literature from the different models of mental illness, and their corresponding models of therapy, provides a rich array of alternatives for organizing people's troubles.

Using our tools from narrative theory, we can say that models of mental illness differentiate themselves through different metaphorical structures. The root metaphors of biopsychiatry, psychoanalysis, or cognitive therapy, for example, all create different ways of perceiving, selecting, and understanding problems. When these different metaphorical structures are put in the context of an individual life, they create very different plot contents for understanding the person's troubles, how those troubles came to be, and how that person might respond to them. These differing metaphors and plot structures go on to create alternative possible narrative identities. The root metaphors people use to understand and plot their troubles become the key elements of who they wish to be. As we discussed in earlier, choosing between different structures of understanding, therefore, is a deeply ethical and political choice. The choice is less about science and "truth" and more about personal preference and affinity. Ultimately, it's a choice about who one wants to become.

Clinicians who are never exposed to narrative theory and never have the option to see narrative theory played out in a literary case example rarely come to appreciate the multiple possibilities for interpreting human troubles or this inescapably ethical dimension of their work. Instead, they tend to work within a single model, or perhaps a couple of models, and to see these models as truth rather than metaphor. If one's model is the truth, then the task is to apply the model, find out what is "really wrong" based on the model, and apply the solution suggested by the model. There's no reason to be curious about other models and no reason to stop and ask, Will this way of organizing this life lead to the kind of narrative identity my client wishes to live? Exposing clinicians to "literary cases" breaks down this kind of clinical dogmatism much more effectively than anything else I have seen. That is why teaching narrative psychiatry always involves two steps—both learning about narrative theory and being able to apply that theory to thick literary case examples that allow that theory to come to life.

With these thoughts in mind, please turn to the appendix at the back of this book to read a copy of the short story "Mrs. Dutta Writes a Letter," by Chitra Divakaruni. Reading the story before proceeding with the next section will be helpful because I will be referring to the story throughout the rest of the book. It is a great story. Enjoy!

Mrs. Dutta's Story as a Literary Case

We can begin the discussion of Mrs. Dutta's story by outlining a basic plot structure. Mrs. Dutta, a widowed woman well over sixty years old, leaves her home in Calcutta and moves to California to live with her son, daughter-in-law, and their two children. Mrs. Dutta's husband died three years earlier, and at the time she decides to leave Calcutta, she feels ready to go and clear that it is the right thing to do. She is so sure of her decision that before leaving she sells the house she and her husband had lived in for forty-five years and gives away all her household effects. Once she is in California, however, conflicts develop with her new life, things do not go well, and she becomes increasingly depressed.

The crisis of the story comes when Mrs. Dutta retreats to her basement bedroom in desperation and despair. The narrator gives a moving description of the depths of her sadness: "In the darkness she lowers herself onto her bed very gently, as though her body were made of the thinnest glass. Or perhaps ice—she is so cold. She sits for a long time with her eyes closed, while inside her head thoughts whirl faster and faster until the disappear in a gray dust storm" (Divakaruni 1999, 46). The story reaches resolution when Mrs. Dutta decides, seemingly against all expectations, to return to Calcutta and live in the spare apartment of one of her oldest friends.

Following a modified version of Tucker's method, I ask narrative psychiatry readers to rewind the story to the moment of crisis. This is the moment when Mrs. Dutta's depression is at its worst and she can no longer go on without making some changes. I ask readers to imagine that Mrs. Dutta comes (or is perhaps brought) to see a narrative psychiatrist at just this moment of crisis. Remember, this is the time in the story before the author has provided a resolution. Indeed, at this moment in the story it is very difficult to imagine how Mrs. Dutta's situation could possibly be resolved. The option of going back to Calcutta does not seem to be viable at that point. Mrs. Dutta seems stuck in her despair.

Imagining a clinical encounter of this kind, we can use it to understand how narrative psychiatry works in clinical practice and how narrative perspectives help conceptualize psychiatric care. Both narrative medicine and narrative psychotherapy suggest that the narrative psychiatrist's first and in many ways foremost task in helping Mrs. Dutta will be getting to know her and developing a rich appreciation of her story. This empathic connection helps Mrs. Dutta become much less alone with her problems and her sadness. She now has a nonjudgmental partner with whom she can share her troubles. Forming this partnership, however, will be only part of the interaction between Mrs. Dutta and the narrative psychiatrist. In addition, Mrs. Dutta will likely want the psychiatrist to recommend an intervention to help her move beyond her current crisis and conflict. Because her problems at this point are relatively mild, the psychiatrist would generally recommend psychotherapy.

But which psychotherapy would a narrative psychiatrist recommend? The marketplace consists of a tremendous variety of options that might be helpful for Mrs. Dutta. And we also have to consider the medication issue. For psychiatrists the therapeutic options include not only psychotherapy but also medications. To make the case even more challenging (and to include the medication dimension), imagine that Mrs. Dutta's depression goes on for a while and gets even worse than it does in the story. In Divakaruni's version of the story, she implies that the abyss of Mrs. Dutta's depression lasts for a only few hours—Mrs. Dutta goes down to her bedroom in her darkest despair and comes back up again a short while later with the resolve to return home. Imagine it happens differently. Imagine that Mrs. Dutta goes down to her bedroom, pulls the covers over her head, sinks further into despair, but this time she is unable to function again for weeks at a time. Imagine this state goes on long enough for Mrs. Dutta to meet the criteria of a *DSM-IV* "Major Depression" with difficulty sleeping, loss of appetite, intense sadness, feelings of worthlessness and hopelessness, and even passive thoughts of suicide.

Now the dilemma becomes even more difficult. When we imagine Mrs. Dutta's depression developing to this point, we open up a panoply of options—ranging from medications to any number of psychotherapy possibilities. How would a narrative psychiatrist proceed in a clinical encounter of this kind? What would he or she recommend for Mrs. Dutta?

Before answering these questions, we need to stay with the dilemma a little longer. It will not do to rush past the conundrums here. We must inhabit the problem more fully to really understand it. To do that, it helps to work through how a range of different therapeutic options could play out for Mrs. Dutta. Otherwise, we tend to lose sight of the fact that there are many options, with different advantages and disadvantages, not simply a best option.

Conclusion

Literary fiction can provide an ideal site for narrative psychiatry case examples because it often gives its readers a thick set of contextual variables from which to understand its characters. In stories of this kind, the meaning of the story is not closed down in advance, and there remain many ways to understand the characters and their dilemmas. When a character's crisis is considered from the perspective of a clinical encounter, students and clinicians can use the story as a tool to develop their capacities for imagining future histories. Clinicians who add a consideration of future history to their previous consideration of present history and past history more easily recognize the storied dimension of clinical work. There is more than one way to tell the story of the past and the present, and those different ways lead to very different future trajectories. The complexity of literary fiction allows clinicians to see this ambiguity of clinical history in the making—past, present, and future.

In the case of Mrs. Dutta, I have used Divakaruni's short story to imagine that Mrs. Dutta brings her problems to a psychiatrist at the height of her troubles. I have imagined that her crisis becomes even worse than it does in the story, to the point that she fits the criteria for a major depression. Before we can offer a future history for Mrs. Dutta, however, we must be patient enough to work through some of her many options. Thus, in the next three chapters I explore in considerable detail how the specific resources of clinical literature and beyond can provide hope and possibility for Mrs. Dutta. The resources I explore in Chapter 6 include mainstream options of biopsychiatry, cognitive-behavioral therapy, and psychoanalysis. Chapter 7 focuses on less common but still mainstream options of interpersonal therapy, family therapy, and humanistic therapy. And Chapter 8 turns to the more alternative resources of spiritual therapy, creative/expressive therapy, and cultural, political, and feminist therapies. For each of these different options, I consider how the narrative elements of metaphor, plot, character, and point of view could play out for Mrs. Dutta. One of the most remarkable aspects of this exercise is how open the story of Mrs. Dutta is to alternative interpretive frames.

CHAPTER SIX

Mainstream Stories I

BIOPSYCHIATRY, COGNITIVE BEHAVIORAL THERAPY, AND PSYCHOANALYSIS

I N THE LAST CHAPTER, I asked readers to imagine Mrs. Dutta, the main character from Chitra Divakaruni's "Mrs. Dutta Writes a Letter," as a potential psychiatric client. Divakaruni carefully and beautifully describes how Mrs. Dutta becomes increasingly sad and hopeless as she realizes the impossibilities of her current living situation. I asked readers to imagine that Mrs. Dutta comes to see a psychiatrist at this time of crisis and that her sadness becomes even worse than in the story, that she becomes so down and despondent she fits the *DSM-IV* criteria of "Major Depression."

In this chapter, we embark on our next creative task with Divakaruni's story—curiously imagining how different clinicians, coming from very different clinical orientations, might respond to Mrs. Dutta. This exercise is invaluable for narrative psychiatrists because narrative work requires more than narrative theory. It also requires a deep appreciation of a variety of clinical and alternative approaches to problems and how these approaches can structure people's narrative identity. The clinical perspectives I explore in this chapter include the mainstream options of biopsychiatry, cognitive behavioral therapy, and psychoanalysis. These are currently the most common clinical perspectives and therefore the ones Mrs. Dutta would most likely encounter. They are also the ones that are easiest to introduce because they are the most well known.

It must be said from the outset that each of these mainstream approaches has its limits and each gives some aspects of a person's life priority over other aspects. Nonetheless, each is important for narrative psychiatry because narrative psychiatry, like all clinical work, is bound by the cultural referent points in which it works. Some of the most important cultural referent points for understanding psychic difference and psychic pain come from the clinical literature. This literature may start in the clinics, but it does not stay there. It moves out into the broader culture to become an important resource for self-understanding. As Tanya Luhrmann puts it, clinical perspectives "seep into popular culture like the dye from a red shirt in hot water" (Luhrmann 2000, 20).

Peter Tyrer and Derek Steinberg's *Models for Mental Disorder* (2005) provides a good introduction to many of the mainstream models of psychiatric thinking, and I use their work to help organize this chapter. Unfortunately, Tyrer and Steinberg, like many similar authors, begin their book with only the barest discussion of the very idea of a "model."[1] Tyrer and Steinberg provide extensive details about differing models but little reflection on the phenomenon of multiple models itself. They brush quickly past questions like what exactly is a "model" and what does it mean that there are multiple models available for psychiatric work? For narrative psychiatry, these theoretical questions are of critical importance. Indeed, non-narrative psychiatry's willingness to dive into clinical details without thinking through the conceptual complexities is what most separates narrative from non-narrative psychiatry.

The conceptual work in earlier chapters gives us a head start for understanding the phenomenon of differing clinical models. Science studies scholars connect the phenomenon of scientific models to the phenomenon of metaphor. A scientific model, they argue, may be understood to be a kind of metaphor. Both scientific models and metaphors organize our thinking by creating an interaction between the unfamiliar and the familiar. Recall how in an earlier example of metaphor, "man is a wolf," men are understood to be more wolflike (and vice versa) after the metaphor is used. Similarly, as Mary Hesse puts it, "Nature becomes more like a machine in the mechanical philosophy, and actual, concrete machines themselves are seen as stripped down to their essential qualities of mass in motion" (Hesse 2000, 351). Scientific models, in other words, function like metaphor by allowing two systems of terms to interact with and adapt to each other.

Science studies scholars rarely have reason to take the next step and link scientific metaphors with lived experience. But this step is essential for narrative psychiatry because the models of mental illness also become important metaphors for living. To connect models of psychiatry with lived experience, it is helpful to follow Paul Ricoeur's path. Ricoeur not only works through the role of metaphor in human understanding but also adds to metaphor the narrative tools of plot and narrative identity. Following Ricoeur, we can say that when models of mental illness seep from the clinic into the culture, they become part of our cultural metaphors of self-experience. In times of trouble, we look through the metaphorical structures of mental models (and other metaphors in our cultural heritage) to perceive, select, and plot aspects of our lives that we believe to be important. These culturally located self stories scaffold our narrative identity and provide us with a compass for living. They tell us where we have been and where we are now, and they provide us with a trajectory into the future.

When narrative clinicians understand multiple models of psychiatry as tools for narrating life stories, they have at their disposal a wealth of resources for helping clients imagine and eventually choose among possible future histories. To understand how models of mental illness can shape narrative identity, it is extremely helpful to see an array of models applied to a single life story—in this case the story of Mrs. Dutta. The exercise is artificial because few clinicians use pure models (most will mix and match in some way), but taking the models one at a time does highlight the way the different models work.

Biopsychiatry

The model of biopsychiatry, or what Tyrer and Steinberg call the "disease model," frames and organizes mental difference through a metaphor of disease (Tyrer and Steinberg 2005, 7). Nobel Prize–winning biopsychiatrist Eric Kandell explains the model this way: "All mental processes, even the most complex psychological processes, derive from operations of the brain. The central tenet of this view is that what we commonly call mind is a range of functions carried out by the brain" (Kandel 1998, 460). Following this metaphorical frame, biopsychiatrists argue that if the brain is the organ of the mind, dysfunctions of mind must therefore be diseases of the brain. "Disease," in this context, means impaired functioning as a consequence of physical and chemical changes. Thus, biopsychiatry has a deep affinity with biomedicine. The only real difference between biomedicine and biopsychiatry is the specificity of the disease. Biomedicine deals with malfunctions that occur in the body, and biopsychiatry deals with malfunctions that generally occur in the nervous system.

Tyrer and Steinberg articulate four principles of a psychiatric disease model:

- Mental pathology is always accompanied by physical pathology
- The classification of this pathology allows mental illness to be classified into different disorders which have characteristic features
- Mental illness is handicapping and biologically disadvantageous
- The cause of mental illness is explicable by its physical consequences (Tyrer and Steinberg 2005, 9)

Following these principles, it makes perfect sense that biopsychiatrist Nancy Andreasen chose to name her best-selling introduction to this model *The Broken Brain* (Andreasen 1984). The term "broken brain" signifies the diseased, or malfunctioning, brain at the core of mental illness.

This term "broken brain" continues to have some purchase in psychiatry and popular culture, but it has gradually been replaced with more ubiquitous phrase "chemical imbalance." Because broken brains cannot usually be demonstrated in individual cases, the phrase "chemical imbalance" has become the popular explanatory metaphor of biopsychiatry. The term is more amorphous than "broken brain," but its implication is more or less the same. In a chemical imbalance, the brain is still broken, just not so broken that you can see it on autopsy or PET scan (or at least not yet). Rather, the brain is broken at the subtle level of chemical functioning. Thus, the signifiers "broken brain" and "chemical imbalance" are perfect sound bite translations of key metaphors of biopsychiatry into everyday language.

For insight into how a biopsychiatrist might perceive Mrs. Dutta's sadness and also how Mrs. Dutta might incorporate that perception into her self-understanding, it is helpful to turn to writings of biopsychiatrists. Donald Klein and Paul Wender's *Understanding Depression: A Complete Guide to Its Diagnosis and Treatment* provides a good example in that these biopsychiatrists tend to use a relatively pure version of the model. They are unusual in that respect, but they are still helpful in terms of seeing the model in operation. Klein and Wender begin their discussion of depression by differentiating mood disorders into major types. They recognize that there is "much confusion about whether these illnesses are produced by psychological experiences or by malfunctioning within the brain (a 'chemical imbalance')" (Klein and Wender 2005, 10). But they assure readers in no uncertain terms that *depression is a disease, a broken brain*. As they put it: "The major point we wish to make is that depression, manic-depression, dysthymic disorder, and cyclothymic disorder are diseases, the product of abnormal biological functioning" (2005, 10).

To make the diagnosis of a specific mood disorder, Klein and Wender use specific diagnostic criteria: "As with any other disease, the physician— the psychiatrist—has guidelines and rules for making the diagnosis" (2005, 10). The diagnostic criteria for depressive disorders involve "the presence or absence of symptoms" over a period of at least two weeks of feeling sad or blue, loss of pleasure, change in eating or sleeping patterns, low energy, being slowed down or restless, limited libido, feeling inadequate or loss of self-worth, less efficiency at work or home, difficulty coping, and poor concentration (2005, 10–12).

Klein and Wender make a point of explaining that the presence of these symptoms indicates a depressive disease regardless of what else is going on in the person's life that may seem like plausible reasons for the sadness. "Life is never perfect," they argue, "and if people look hard enough, they can find some reason for feeling bad. Even a major loss, such as a death in the family or a divorce, may not be the real reason for your depressed emotional state" (2005, 13). For Klein and Wender, depressive disease is "often triggered by a real event—the death of a loved one, for example— but still requires treatment" as a disease (2005, 13). Furthermore, because depressive disease makes it more difficult for people to function, depression itself is often the cause of life stresses "such as the loss of a job or the breakup of a relationship" (2005, 13). This means that what looks like contextual precipitating events for depressive symptoms may actually be the result of the depressive disease itself.

If Mrs. Dutta were to see a biopsychiatrist like Klein or Wender, how would he or she interpret Mrs. Dutta's troubles? What elements of Mrs. Dutta's life would the clinician focus on, and what course of future action would he or she suggest? Based on Klein and Wender's descriptions, a biopsychiatrist would first listen to Mrs. Dutta's story with an ear and an eye out for signs and symptoms of mental disease. The biopsychiatrist would have several findings right away. Mrs. Dutta is easily tearful (Divakaruni

1999, 31),[2] she is wracked with "doubt" (35), and she has waves of "anger" and "shame" (32). These waves of emotion are sometimes so intense that they create a "burning, acid and indigestible" sensation that "coats her throat in molten metal" (32). Mrs. Dutta has become sad to the point that, when asked if she is happy, she develops deep "insidious feelings" of despair (31). Also, when asked about her previous home in Calcutta, Mrs. Dutta relates that she sometimes feels so sad it is "like someone has reached in and torn a handful of [her] chest" (33). In addition, she has feelings of "heaviness" that "pull at her entire body" (33), and, although it may be related to past sleeping patterns, she seems to have signs of early morning awakening (29).

All these symptoms are so severe that they have resulted in a marked drop in Mrs. Dutta's functioning. Mrs. Dutta is clearly a capable woman who has managed a large household in the past, but she is currently having difficulty coping at her son's house even though she has few responsibilities. In addition, Mrs. Dutta has a history of depression. She had similar episode several months earlier after getting pneumonia (34, 35). At that time, she became so depressed and hopeless she felt she had "no reason to get well" (35). If we add to these findings our imaginary additional ones of several weeks in bed more or less nonfunctional, with deepening feelings of sadness and despair, and with passive thoughts of suicide, then it seems clear that a biopsychiatrist would diagnose Mrs. Dutta with a major depression, or what Klein and Wender frequently call a "biological depression" (Klein and Wender 2005, 46).

After making the diagnosis, the psychiatrist would meet with Mrs. Dutta and perhaps her family to explain her findings. The psychiatrist would make it clear that depression is a common illness that is treatable and that no one is to blame for this problem. Biological depression, the psychiatrist would emphasize, is a disease like any other disease. Researchers, the psychiatrist would go on, are making great progress in understanding the brain pathology involved, and, although this is an oversimplification, we now know that depression is caused by a kind of chemical imbalance in the brain. If Mrs. Dutta or a family member asked about the significance of her recent move to the United States and the loss of her home, the psychiatrist would carefully point out that these kinds of environmental factors are not sufficient to explain Mrs. Dutta's condition any more than if Mrs. Dutta had the medical diagnoses of high blood pressure or diabetes. There are millions of people in today's globalized world who move back and forth between different countries without falling into depression.

Using Klein and Wender's book as a guide, we can get an idea of the treatment the psychiatrist would suggest for Mrs. Dutta. The psychiatrist would explain that in cases of biological depression "treatment with medications should usually be the first choice" (Klein and Wender 2005, 46). The psychiatrist would then explain that although antidepressants can be helpful, "these drugs often take three to four weeks to work" (2005, 47). She or he would further explain that Mrs. Dutta will need to "continue on the medication for at least six months and that she would need regular checkups during this period" (2005, 47). These checkups would be similar to visits to a medical doctor, brief sessions of fifteen to twenty minutes to review Mrs. Dutta's progress and make any needed changes or adjustments in her medications. The biopsychiatrist would be optimistic that Mrs. Dutta will have a good recovery on medications. As Klein and Wender put it, "Biological treatments for depression are dramatically effective. Eighty percent, or even more, of individuals suffering from a major depression will respond to one or another of the antidepressant drugs, singly or in combination" (2005, 101).

Many biopsychiatrists suggest combining medication with psychotherapy, but if Mrs. Dutta's psychiatrist used a purer biomedical model similar to that of Klein and Wender, she or he would likely advise against psychotherapy. Klein and Wender make it clear that they do not believe psychotherapies are much more effective than "brief consultations with a physician who follows no specific psychotherapeutic approach" (2005, 102). And they argue that trials of psychotherapy can often be demoralizing because if patients do not get better they can feel blamed for their problems, as if they are not working hard enough. "They may even conclude that they are not 'good patients' and become more depressed" (2005, 104). Thus, for Klein and Wender, "it seems reasonable to start with medication since it is faster and cheaper and avoids the frustration a biologically depressed person experiences in psychotherapy" (2005, 104).

If Mrs. Dutta stays in treatment with a biopsychiatrist like Klein or Wender and if she internalizes this perspective, the narrative outcome for Mrs. Dutta will be that she will adopt a narrative identity as a mental patient. She will understand herself as having a biological vulnerability to depression, and she will restory the events of her life within the metaphors of biological psychiatry. She will see the difficulties she is having at her new home as caused by the disease of depression, and she will work with the psychiatrist to treat her disease through monitoring its signs and symptoms and making adjustments in her medications. If one medication does not work or works only part way, she will try other medications or perhaps a combination of medications. If her situation gets worse, she may be hospitalized and perhaps treated with ECT. If her depression becomes chronic, she and her psychiatrist will look for a more intense treatment setting, like a day hospital or perhaps supportive living. If she makes progress, her medications may be reduced or perhaps gradually discontinued. But even if that does happen, Mrs. Dutta's identity as a mental patient will continue, and she will know that if her symptoms return she will need to restart medical treatments.

Cognitive Behavioral Therapy

The cognitive behavioral model of mental suffering shifts the focus from "broken brains" to what we could call "broken thoughts" or "broken thinking." The basic metaphorical frame of this model is that errors and distortions in thinking lead to mental illness. Tyrer and Steinberg describe four central tenants of the cognitive behavioral model:

- People's view of their world is determined by their thinking (cognition)
- Cognition influences symptoms, behavior and attitudes and therefore the main features of mental illness
- The persistence of mental illness is a consequence of continuing errors in thinking and maladaptive behaviors that become reinforcing
- Significant change in mental disorder is always associated with significant change in cognition and behavior (Tyrer and Steinberg 2005, 76)

An example of the connection between cognition and psychiatric symptoms would be a person who views a situation as threatening and then feels tremendous anxiety. Another example would be a person who views his or her troubles as overwhelming and hopeless and then feels extremely depressed. The founder of this model, Aaron Beck, puts it this way, "Cognitive theory is based on the assumption that the way individuals interpret their experiences has significant impact on their emotions and actions—indeed, on their overall psychological functioning" (Beck and Newman 2005, 2596).

Cognitive behavioral therapy (CBT) takes this model of mental suffering and turns it into specific strategies and techniques of therapy. The most important strategy of CBT involves setting up a therapeutic relationship in which the therapist and patient explore the person's cognitive processes together and try to modify them. Beck recommends a therapeutic approach he calls "collaborative empiricism," which views the patient as a kind of practical scientist who needs help correcting a faulty hypothesis about his or her life (Beck, Rush, Shaw, and Emery. 1979, 6). The therapeutic techniques used in this process are both cognitive and behavioral. The cognitive techniques focus on "identifying and testing the patient's beliefs, exploring their origins and basis, correcting them if they fail an empirical or logical test, or problem solving" (Beck and Weishaar 2005, 240). The behavioral techniques involve a variety of procedures such as daily activities schedules, mastery and pleasure ratings, graded tasks, role-play, and assertiveness practice.

If Mrs. Dutta were to see a cognitive behavioral therapist, the therapist would likely be impressed with the power of cognitive theory to explain Mrs. Dutta's depression. Even in the early stages of Mrs. Dutta's troubles there is a clear link between her thoughts and her sadness. The link goes back in the story to the time when Mrs. Dutta was still in Calcutta living on her own and became ill with pneumonia. The experience of being ill while living alone was very different from the prior experience she had while living with her husband and children. In prior times, Mrs. Dutta's family constantly nagged her to do this and do that and to hurry up and get better. But this time she was under no pressure to get better, "no one's life was inconvenienced the least by her illness," and it seemed that she "had no reason to get well."

Remarkably, as soon as Mrs. Dutta had the thought that it did not matter whether she got better, her depressive symptoms began. As the narrator of the story puts it, "*When this thought occurred* to Mrs. Dutta, she was so frightened that her body grew numb. The walls of the room spun into blackness: the bed on which she lay, a vast four-poster she had shared with Sagar's father since their wedding, rocked like a dinghy caught in a storm: a great hollow roaring reverberated inside her head. For a moment, unable to move or see, she thought, *I'm dead*" (35; first italics added).

Thus, from early on, there is a clear connection between Mrs. Dutta's thoughts and her mood. For the cognitive therapist, Mrs. Dutta's sadness during her time in Calcutta would be related to several information-processing errors, or "cognitive distortions," typically seen in depression. Mrs. Dutta's cognitive distortions included overgeneralization, magnification, and personalization (Beck et al. 1979, 14). She overgeneralized from the thought that her family no longer needs her to the idea that she is no longer needed at all. She magnified the meaning of the thought to a catastrophe. And she personalized the situation to blame herself as being somehow unworthy of being needed.

Mrs. Dutta's cognitive therapist would likely conclude that Mrs. Dutta was able to briefly escape these thoughts by moving to the United States. But once Mrs. Dutta arrived in the United States, the thoughts reappeared, and she gradually sank further into the classic "cognitive triad" of depression (Beck et al. 1979, 10). Caught in this cognitive triad, Mrs. Dutta developed dysfunctionally negative views of (1) herself, (2) her life experience (the world in general), and (3) her sense of the future. Mrs. Dutta's self-worth deteriorated as she came to believe she had nothing to offer her family. She increasingly felt that her grandchildren were not interested in learning about their heritage, nor were they interested in the food she cooks (35, 33). She also had great trouble doing simple things like running the washing machine or understanding the jokes on television (35, 29), and she blamed herself for her son and daughter-in-law's marriage problems (45). In addition, she came to view the United States as a hopelessly alien world, with strange customs and values, where the rules are mixed up and "upside down" (35, 36, 44). As she sank further into this negative image of herself and the world, Mrs. Dutta became bleak about her future and unable to see hope for improvement. In the end, even going across the street to meet the neighbor seemed impossible (41).

Mrs. Dutta's therapist would recommend CBT for her depression and would explain that the standard duration of treatment is fifteen to twenty sessions over a twelve-week period. The therapist would add that this time frame can vary from person to person and in practice CBT may go on considerably longer. The therapist would then work with Mrs. Dutta to set up the goals of the therapy and would likely initiate early behavioral techniques. Mrs. Dutta might be asked to complete a Daily Activities Schedule (DAS) to give the therapist information about how she is spending (or misspending) her time. For example, too much time sitting and worrying would be seen as a pattern likely to be "low in pleasure or mastery" and would predictably keep Mrs. Dutta "mired in helplessness and hopelessness" (Beck and Newman 2005, 2600). Mrs. Dutta and the therapist would use the DAS to identify behavioral problems and set behavioral goals. They might, for example, agree on prospectively scheduling activities that help mobilize Mrs. Dutta, thus "counteracting depressogenic inertia" (2005, 2600). These activities would be increased in small gradual steps and through graded-task assignments.

In addition, Mrs. Dutta would be taught to monitor her automatic negative thoughts and learn to evaluate these thoughts in a critical but nonjudgmental manner. As Mrs. Dutta used the therapy to view her thoughts more objectively, she would clarify and modify the meanings she assigned to events. Through collaborative empiricism, Mrs. Dutta and the therapist would work to produce cognitive shifts that would create a "boost in morale" and "improved hopefulness" (2005, 2601). Mrs. Dutta would be shown how, by changing her thoughts, she can change her mood, feel better, and cope more effectively. The therapist might also teach Mrs. Dutta to hypothesize reasonable responses to her automatic thoughts through Socratic questions designed to improve her reality testing. By asking herself Socratic questions Mrs. Dutta could learn to think "logically, flexibly, and hopefully" (2005, 2601). Typical Socratic questions include:

- "What are some other plausible ways I can look at this situation?"
- "What concrete, factual evidence supports or refutes my automatic thoughts?"
- "Realistically, what is the worst thing that can happen in this situation, and would I be able to live through it? What is the best thing that could happen? Now that I have considered both extremes, neither of which is statistically likely to occur, what is the most likely outcome of this situation?"
- "What constructive action can I take to deal with this situation?"

- "What are the pros and cons of maintaining my automatic thoughts as they are?

- "What sincere, helpful, realistic advice would I give to a good friend in the same situation?" (2005, 2601)

For example, Mrs. Dutta might state that she sees no reason to try understanding American television because the reference points are too foreign, she will fail, and she will end up feeling worse. This prediction would be viewed by Mrs. Dutta's therapist as a hypothesis. She would encourage Mrs. Dutta to test the hypothesis by trying to concentrate on the television, seeing for herself how much she is able to comprehend, and rating her moods during and after the fact. This procedure would be considered a "win-win proposition" in that Mrs. Dutta would "transcend a state of inertia and helplessness simply by virtue of testing the hypothesis, regardless of whether she exceeds her expectations in the process" (2005, 2601).

There is some evidence in the story that Mrs. Dutta might appreciate this kind of approach. There are several moments when she spontaneously monitors and corrects her thoughts without exposure to CBT. For example, when Mrs. Dutta finds herself feeling bitter about the way her grandchildren treat her, she corrects her thoughts by telling herself that "holding on to grudges is too exhausting" (32). When she finds herself longing for Calcutta, she tells herself "only fools indulge in nostalgia" (33). When she has a deeply critical thought about her past life, she works hard to "erase such an insidious idea from her mind" (44). And, in a letter to her friend Roma, she spontaneously reframes her struggles with the United States as "I'm fitting in so well here, you'd never guess I came only two months back. I've found new ways of doing things, of solving problems creatively. You would be most proud of me" (38). All these spontaneous efforts at cognitive therapy suggest that Mrs. Dutta might value her work in CBT.

If she did, the narrative outcome of CBT for Mrs. Dutta is that she would come to understand her depression as related to her cognitive distortions. Her therapist would be clear that these cognitive distortions are not the cause of her mental illness. Causality in CBT is best understood in "terms of the complex interactions of innate biological, developmental, and environmental (including interpersonal) factors" (Beck and Newman

2005, 2597). But even if her cognitions do not cause her depression, they remain an effective entry point for intervention and correction. Through her work in CBT, Mrs. Dutta would recognize that she can control her moods if she can control her thoughts. She would learn multiple skills for doing this and would practice implementing these skills. If Mrs. Dutta developed a return of symptoms, she would know she can always return to CBT for a booster and refresher. Thus, in the end, the narrative outcome for Mrs. Dutta's is that through CBT she will understand that her moods are ultimately up to her and the amount of effort she devotes to monitoring and modifying her maladaptive thinking.

Psychoanalysis

The psychoanalytic model, often called the "psychodynamic model," is less clearly demarcated than biopsychiatry or cognitive behaviorism, and there are many different schools of psychoanalysis. Psychoanalysis should therefore be seen as a collection of models rather than a single model, depending on which school of psychoanalysis one emphasizes. As Tyrer and Steinberg point out, however, there are clear similarities between various psychoanalytic models, and there are basic assumptions common to most psychodynamic therapies (Tyrer and Steinberg 2005, 42).

The leading assumption for psychodynamic therapists is that problematic patterns of feeling lead to difficulties being in the world. These patterns of feelings are complicated, inconsistent, and often in conflict with one another. A person's most intense feeling patterns often arise in childhood during interactions with caretakers and significant others. Although these early feelings may be understandable at the time they arise, they are often much less understandable later in life. The transference of these intense feelings from childhood on to current situations causes most of the problems. People repeatedly fall into a repetition of old feelings because these patterns of feelings are so ingrained and second nature that the history of these feelings is often unconscious. Even the fact that the person is having idiosyncratic reactions to the world is outside his or her awareness. As Tyrer and Steinberg put it, "What the patient is aware of, or an attitude he or she adopts, is the tip of the iceberg of feelings, much of which is only partially conscious, or unconscious, but which is influential nonetheless" (2005, 43).

Thus, what we could call the unifying metaphorical frame or core model of psychoanalysis is that there is significant "mental activity continuing outside our awareness, yet at the same time being able to influence" our experiences (2005, 45). This idea goes against the grain of our basic intuitions and common sense. People tend to perceive their feelings as natural reactions to their current situation rather than complicated markers of their history with the world, or, worse, as the tip of the iceberg of a whole series of additional and often contradictory feelings.

Psychodynamic therapists focus their attention on these patterns of unconscious feelings much more than symptoms or *DSM-IV* diagnostic categories because they see unconscious feelings as more important than the particular symptoms. From a psychodynamic perspective, if you treat the manifest symptoms without addressing the underlying patterns and feelings, new symptoms will simply emerge. Instead of making specific diagnoses based on manifest symptoms, the task of psychoanalysis is to tap into unconscious feelings through the process of therapy and bring these feelings to the light of awareness. If a person can use the therapeutic situation to gain insight into these feelings and work through the intensity of their original causes, she or he has a good chance of responding differently to them and avoiding painful repetition with the corresponding heartache.

Out of the many models of depression within psychoanalysis, the work of George Pollock is particularly applicable to Mrs. Dutta's situation.[3] Pollock builds on Sigmund Freud's classic "Mourning and Melancholia" and the history of psychoanalytic work since Freud to develop an understanding of depression as pathological mourning. For Pollock, mourning is a necessary adaptation process that allows humans to successfully cope with the losses of life. Death of a loved one, or what Pollock calls bereavement, is just one of the many losses that may elicit a mourning process. In addition to death, the loss of anything that people are attached to can initiate mourning—whether it be marital separation, divorce, loss of support systems, job loss, serious illness of family members, serious surgical procedures, aging, and so on.

Once mourning begins, the person can expect to go through a series of phases and stages in which the loss is metabolized. These stages are often painful and involve waves of intense emotional desire to be back with the person, place, or thing that has been lost. Being with these painful emotions is what Freud called "the work of mourning." For most people, it takes considerable time and emotional support to successfully complete the mourning process, and there is no guarantee that people will come to the other side of mourning. Incomplete mourning or mourning gone awry can leave traces that disturb the person for the rest of his or her lifetime.

Pollock refers to four possible outcomes of mourning:

1. "Normal" or successful resolution which results in "creative activity, creative reinvested living, creative products."
2. "Arrestation" of the mourning process with continued denial of the loss and the inability to give up the attachment.
3. "Fixations" to earlier developmental stages which are reactivated by incomplete mourning.
4. "Pathological" or "deviated" mourning processes that are variously diagnosed by mental health providers as depression or depressive states (Pollock 1978, 273).

The most successful outcome of mourning "involves not only detachment from internal representations and external absences, but reattachments and freedom (i.e., liberation) at the concluding adaptation" (Pollock 1989, xiii). Pollock refers to this as a process of "mourning-liberation" to emphasis the two mutually related dynamics of mourning—letting go and reattachment. For people who are unable to process their losses, they may find themselves falling into any of the three alternative outcomes to mourning.

If Mrs. Dutta saw a psychodynamic therapist who worked with Pollock's model of depression, the therapist would likely suspect some form of pathological grieving. The therapist would understand the power and intensity of this unresolved grief as largely outside Mrs. Dutta's awareness. Still, this unconscious grief would provide a good explanation of her symptoms of depression. There are many aspects of Mrs. Dutta's story that the therapist would pick up on that would lead her or him to this conclusion. Mrs. Dutta expresses great nostalgia for her home in Calcutta and for the life she had when her family was all together. She is extremely sad about leaving India and attached to news from home (31). She misses the street life of Calcutta (39), the crowded living conditions (40), her many friends and especially her closest confident, Roma (39). She longs for the home that she had lived in for more than forty years, her maid (39), and even her Calcutta kitchen with its new stove, brass pots, meat safe, and mouthwatering spices (39). As Mrs. Dutta explains to Roma, "I miss it all so much. Sometimes I feel like someone has reached in and torn a handful of my chest" (33).

In addition, Mrs. Dutta mourns for the time when her family was all together. She longs for the closeness of that time, the pranks her son used to pull (30), the way he used to crawl into her bed when there was a monsoon (30), the daily "sleep-warm clasp" of mornings with her husband (28), and the way her husband used to play tricks on the children (42). She longs for the role she had in the family, where she had purpose and was important. Mrs. Dutta hoped to reconstitute that role by moving to the United States but gradually has had to accept that she cannot play that role again. She used to get up early, to prepare the family for their day, but now she is told that she must not get up so early because it wakes everyone up (30). She imagined that she would teach her grandchildren about their heritage, but it turns out they would rather watch television (32). She hoped to cook "proper Indian food" for the family with "puffed-up chapatis, fish curry in mustard sauce and real pulao with raisins and cashews and ghee," but finds out that her daughter-in-law does not like the fat and her grandchildren prefer burritos from the freezer and Rice-a-Roni (33). In short, Mrs. Dutta has no meaningful contribution, and she yearns for that "sweet aching urgency of being needed again" (33). When she thinks of these disappointments, heaviness pulls at her entire body (33).

On hearing these signs of Mrs. Dutta's unresolved mourning, the psychodynamic therapist would likely suggest psychoanalytically oriented psychotherapy sessions once or twice a week with no specific end point. Mrs. Dutta would be asked to use the sessions to talk about her feelings during the week and during the sessions. She would be asked not to censure these feelings and to be as true to their expression as she possibly can—even if the feelings are uncomfortable, or painful, or in some way taboo. The therapist would explain that his or her role is to listen with Mrs. Dutta, to help facilitate her expression of her feelings, and to provide suggestions and insight where he or she could.

If all went well, Mrs. Dutta would use the support of the therapy sessions to feel the full intensity of her grief, to gain insight into the power of these feelings, to restart the mourning process, and to work through these feelings of loss. In all likelihood, the feelings of attachment and loss would also play themselves out with the therapist as well. During their work together, the therapist would help Mrs. Dutta connect her current griefs during and outside therapy to unresolved griefs from earlier in her life. Although we do not know a great deal of detail about Mrs. Dutta's early years, we do know that at age seventeen she was moved abruptly from her childhood family to her husband's family. This move was the result of an arranged marriage, and from what we have in the story, it does not sound like she was able to fully process that loss. It may well be that Mrs. Dutta's unresolved mourning may go back much further than those losses in her adult life and that they may repeat earlier feelings from her relations with her parents and caregivers.

Over time, Mrs. Dutta would use psychodynamic therapy to let go of these many attachments and free up emotional energy to reattach to new possibilities in her new life. If Pollock is correct, the clinical outcome of this process would not only ameliorate Mrs. Dutta's depression but also lead to a period of increased creativity and heightened vitality. But regardless of the clinical outcome, the narrative outcome would be that Mrs. Dutta would likely come to understand her depression and sadness in the context of the many losses of her life. She would give meaning to her troubles through this narrative of loss. She would be less likely to see herself as having a biological depression and more likely to see herself as a victim of her situation. This would provide a future direction for her in the sense that she would see her task as continued work on unresolved grief and ongoing efforts to make new attachments.

Conclusion

Biopsychiatry, cognitive-behavioral therapy, and psychodynamic therapy are all effective for understanding Mrs. Dutta's sadness. Each model works like a metaphor to select from Mrs. Dutta's life specific variables of attention and priority. Biopsychiatry selects for biological symptoms, cognitive-behavioral therapy selects for cognitive distortions, and psychoanalysis selects for unconscious conflicts. Mrs. Dutta's sadness readily lends itself to a consideration of any of these sets of variables. If Mrs. Dutta were to work with a clinician using one of these models, she would learn to plot her life consistent with the particular model. She would gain a historical explanation of her sadness and specific strategies of intervention going forward. In addition, this metaphorical and plot structure would become a significant feature of her narrative identification. By recognizing the diversity of options among these three mainstream models, narrative psychiatrists move beyond narrative theory to develop a deeper understanding of the particulars of psychiatric experience. But, as we will see in the next two chapters, these three models are only the beginning of Mrs. Dutta's narrative options.

CHAPTER SEVEN

Mainstream Stories II

INTERPERSONAL THERAPY, FAMILY THERAPY, AND HUMANISTIC THERAPY

T HIS CHAPTER CONSIDERS the narrative resources for Mrs. Dutta of a group of therapies that, while still in the mainstream, are less common than the big three of the last chapter. These approaches include interpersonal therapy, family therapy, and humanistic therapy.

Interpersonal Therapy

The model of suffering adopted by interpersonal psychotherapy makes an important shift from the models we have discussed thus far. Interpersonal psychotherapy moves the focus from the individual person to the person's interpersonal context. The founder of interpersonal psychotherapy, Gerald Klerman, associates the emergence of this approach with the pioneering work Harry Stack Sullivan (Klerman, Weissman, Rounsaville, and Chevron 1984, 6). The epigraph to Klerman and his associate's first major book on interpersonal therapy comes from Sullivan and gives a good sense of this change of focus: "The field of psychiatry is the field of interpersonal relations, under any and all circumstances . . . a personality can never be isolated from the complex of interpersonal relations in which the person lives and has his being" (1984, v). Sullivan developed this social turn for psychiatry because, although he first trained in psychoanalysis, he also studied widely in social theory and social science. Indeed, throughout much of his career he argued that clinical psychiatry should be closely linked to anthropology, sociology, and social psychology.

The interpersonal model that grew out of Sullivan's work focuses therapeutic attention to the micro social relations of family, romantic ties, friendships, and coworkers. From an interpersonal perspective, the most important variables for understanding and intervening in human troubles do not reside in the person's head—whether those variables are conceptualized as neurochemical imbalances, cognitive distortions, or unconscious patterns of feeling. The most important variables reside in the person's close and frequent social interactions with others.

For interpersonal psychotherapy, this move to the interpersonal level is not a theory of causation. Unlike some social models, interpersonal psychotherapists do not make the assumption that the causes of mental illness are located in the social environment. However, and this is crucial, "interpersonal psychotherapy does assume that the development and maintenance of some psychiatric illnesses occur in a social and interpersonal context and that the onset, response to treatment, and outcomes are influenced by the interpersonal relations between the patient and significant others" (Wilfley 2005, 2610).

Klerman and associates used this interpersonal model to work out a detailed approach to depression. This approach focused on maladaptive interpersonal settings in which the depression develops and is maintained. The four social domains that interpersonal psychotherapy considers are grief, interpersonal role disputes, role transitions, and interpersonal deficits. Interpersonal psychotherapy's concern with grief is similar to that discussed by Pollock in his mourning-liberation theory, and this part of the interpersonal approach was inspired by much of the same psychoanalytic work that inspired Pollock. The main difference is that interpersonal psychotherapy focuses relatively less on the interpsychic aspects of grief and more on its interpersonal dimensions. Interpersonal psychotherapy tends to focus specifically on the death or loss of significant others (as opposed to broader losses). Plus, interpersonal therapy takes a much more behavioral approach that encourages people to fill the "empty space" lost by loved ones. For example, interpersonal therapists will likely be "very active in leading the patient to consider various alternative ways (dating, church, organizations, work) to become involved with others again" (Klerman, Weissman, Rounsaville, and Chevron 1984, 101).

The next three areas of attention are clearly devoted to the interpersonal domain. Interpersonal role disputes "are conflicts with a significant other (e.g., a partner, other family member, coworker, or close friend) that emerge from differences in expectations about the relationship" (Wilfley

2005, 2610). Role transitions are "difficulties associated with a change in life status (e.g., graduation, leaving a job, moving, marriage/divorce, retirement, change in health status)" (2005, 2610). And interpersonal deficits are patterns of difficulty throughout a person's life finding and keeping sustaining relationships. Patients with interpersonal deficits usually have a history of social isolated or have chronically unfulfilling relationships.

The strategies and techniques of interpersonal psychotherapy (ITP) bear some resemblance to the medical model, to CBT, and to psychodynamic psychotherapy. In many ways, one could see ITP as a hybrid approach that includes techniques from all of these domains. Like the medical model, ITP emphasizes the importance of establishing a psychiatric diagnosis and giving the patient the sick role. Different from the medical model, ITP justifies psychiatric diagnosis and the sick role largely for social reasons: "Consistent with the medical model, receiving a formal diagnosis reinforces the idea that the patient has a known condition that can be treated . . . [and is] designed to temporarily exempt the individual from other responsibilities so as to devote full attention to recovery" (Wilfley 2005, 2612). That said, ITP therapists do include biological variables as possible factors in causation and they are comfortable with medication treatments alongside psychotherapeutic approaches.

Similar to CBT, interpersonal therapy tends to be short term and highly structured. Therapy generally lasts 12 to 20 sessions over a 4- to 5-month period. The initial phase is devoted to identifying target areas. Intermediate work is devoted to problem solving in the target areas. The termination phase consolidates gains and prepares the patient for future work on their own. Similar to psychodynamic approaches, IPT appreciates the importance of unconscious processes such as unresolved anger or defense mechanisms like "projection, denial, isolation, undoing, or repression" (Klerman, Weissman, Rounsaville, and Chevron 1984, 15). But, in IPT, the therapist does not see these phenomena as signs of internal conflict as much as blocks to interpersonal relations.

If Mrs. Dutta saw an interpersonal psychotherapist, her therapist would diagnose depression and recommend individual psychotherapy. The therapist would begin with an "interpersonal inventory," and she would develop of an "interpersonal formulation" of Mrs. Dutta's sadness (Wilfley 2005, 2611). This interpersonal formulation would link Mrs. Dutta's psychiatric symptoms to the four interpersonal problem areas discussed above. The therapist would likely be impressed with the relevance of interpersonal theory for explaining Mrs. Dutta's troubles. Mrs. Dutta has unresolved grief issues related to the death of her husband and the loss of her friend Roma. She has interpersonal role disputes surrounding conflicting expectations in the new family, and she has role transition problems associated with the recent changes in her life status. Fortunately, however, Mrs. Dutta does not have a significant history of interpersonal deficits and her current interpersonal problems seem relatively recent. For the interpersonal therapist, this would be considered a good prognostic sign.

The goal of the therapist would be to reduce Mrs. Dutta's social isolation by helping her "enhance the quality of existing relationships and encouraging the formation of new relationships" (2005, 2613). Should Mrs. Dutta stay with the therapist and adopt her model, the narrative outcome would be that she would come to understand her sadness as a kind of loneliness. Mrs. Dutta would see that a series of events came together in her life to leave her isolated and alone. She would appreciate that just as a plant without water would understandably wilt, a person without interpersonal connections would understandably feel sad. Mrs. Dutta would recognize that although her isolation cannot completely explain her depression, reducing this isolation is the most powerful step toward alleviating depression. As Mrs. Dutta makes progress along this interpersonal path, she would likely feel better. If not, if she is unable to enhance her relationships and make new ones, she would understand the need for more intensive methods—such as a day program or supported living.

Family Therapy

Like interpersonal therapy, family therapy views people's problems in the context of their relational interactions. But, different from interpersonal approaches, family therapy focuses attention more specifically on the family and it intervenes with the family as a whole "to identify and change problematic, maladaptive, self-defeating, repetitive relationship patterns" (Goldenberg and Goldenberg 2005, 372). Family therapy conceptualizes the symptomatic family member not as the primary patient, but as the "identified patient." The shift from "patient" to "identified patient" marks how family therapy sees the family system itself—not the individual—as the primary unit of treatment. The identified patient may have the most obvious troubles, but he or she is viewed as a "symptom bearer, express-ing the family's disequilibrium or current dysfunction" rather than the source of the problem (2005, 372).

Family therapists sometimes compare and contrast the more common individual approaches to their interpersonal approach through a trans-portation metaphor. If individually oriented therapists are like mechanics, family therapists are like traffic engineers. The mechanic is concerned with "the internal working of vehicles" (Barker 1986, 1). Where as the traffic engineer's job is to "see that vehicles travel smoothly on highways" without bunching up into traffic jams or, worse, wrecking into each other due to poor planning and problematic traffic patterns. From a family therapy perspective, "a well functioning family system helps the develop-ment and adjustment of the family members, just as traffic runs more smoothly in a well-designed and efficient road system than in a poor sys-tem" (1986, 1). This transportation metaphor helps explain why many fam-ily therapists tend to be "present centered" and to "examine here-and-now interactions rather than look to history for antecedent causes" (Becvar and Becvar 2003, 10). From the perspective of a traffic engineer, the road sys-tem's history matters less than innovative ways to get traffic flowing again.

Family therapy has multiple and complex historical roots. It most clearly begins in the 1950s with multigenerational research by Murray Bowen, Jay Haley, Don Jackson, Carl Whitaker, and Lyman Wynne into psychosis and schizophrenia. In addition, Nathan Ackerman and Salva-dor Minuchin's family work with child and adolescent problems begins during the same time period. These first-generation family therapists were deeply critical of prevailing approaches to human troubles. They all "had in common a passionate questioning of the dominant individual models (primarily psychoanalytic) of problem development, maintenance, and treatment and an assertion of the explanatory power of thinking in terms of circular (versus linear) causality" (Gurman and Lebow 2005, 2587).

The tension between family therapy and individual therapy has dissi-pated over time, but family therapists still consider the distinction between linear and circular causality to be the basis of the very different world view of family therapy (Becvar and Becvar 2003, 3). The linear worldview of most therapies believes that "event A causes event B in a linear (unidirec-tional) fashion." If asked, why did B happen, the linear answer would be "because A did such and such" (2003, 4). Family therapists, by contrast, rely on systems theory and cybernetics worldview which makes this linear thinking untenable and tends to emphasize circular concepts like "reciprocity, recursion, and shared responsibility." For family therapist, "A and B exist in the context of a relationship in which each influences the other and both are equally cause and effect of each other's behavior" (2003, 10). This systems perspective is holistic rather than reductive and the focus is "on the process, or context, that gives meaning to the events instead of only on the individuals or the events in isolation" (2003, 10).

Several schools of family therapy have developed over time, but they all have considerable common ground. Irene and Herbert Goldenberg point to several basic premises:

1. People are products of their social connections, and attempts to help them must take family relationships into account.
2. Symptomatic behavior in an individual arises from a context of relationships, and interventions to help that person are most effective when those faulty interactive patters are altered.
3. Individual symptoms are maintained externally in current family systems transactions.
4. Conjoint sessions in which the family is the therapeutic unit and the focus is on family interaction are more effective in producing change than attempts to uncover intrapsychic problems in individuals by therapy via individual sessions.
5. Assessing family subsystems and the permeability of boundaries within the family and between the family and the outside world offers important clues regarding family organization and susceptibility to change.
6. Traditional psychiatric diagnostic labels based on individual psychopathology fail to provide an understanding of family dysfunctions and tend to pathologize individuals.
7. The goal of family therapy is to change maladaptive or dysfunctional family interactive patterns. (Goldenberg and Goldenberg 2005, 386–87)

All of these common features focus on a systems frame of reference. Family therapists, in other words, view the family as an ongoing living organism. They see the family as a "complexly organized, durable, causal network of related parts that together constitute and entity larger than the simple sum of its individual members" (2005, 373). Accordingly, family therapists pay close attention to two basic aspects of family organization: "structure" and "process."

Structure refers to how a family "arranges, organizes, and maintains itself at a particular cross section of time" (2005, 373). The three structural systems that family therapists most address are the spousal, parental, and sibling subsystems. The spousal subsystem is considered especially important for a family because "any dysfunction in the spousal subsystem is bound to reverberate throughout the family, resulting in scapegoating of [other family members] or co-opting them into alliances with one spouse against the other" (2005, 375). Family therapists also pay close attention to the structural question of "boundaries," which are "invisible lines that separate a system, a subsystem, or an individual from outside surroundings" (2005, 375). Rigid boundaries are overly restrictive and prevent little movement across them. Diffuse boundaries, by contrast, are overly blurred and porous. "Excessively rigid boundaries characterize *disengaged families* in which members feel isolated from one another, while diffuse boundaries identify *enmeshed families* in which members are intertwined in one another's lives" (2005, 375).

Process refers to the way a family "evolves, adapts, or changes over time" (2005, 373). Based on the cybernetic principle of feedback loops, family therapists understand families as seeking homeostasis. In times of stress, families try to maintain or regain a stable environment "by activating family-learned mechanisms to decrease the stress or restore internal balance" (2005, 274). However, families must not only maintain their equilibrium but also adapt to inevitable life changes. Typical changes that affect the American family "life cycle" include marriage, new children, the shifts of adolescence and young adult children, and failing health and death (Kaslow, Dausch, and Celano 2003, 406). For immigrant families, they often face additional changes associated with adapting to a new country. These changes put considerable pressure on the "nature and structure of relationships across generations, based on the interface of their new culture with cultural patterns from their country of origin" (2003, 406).

Structure and process come together through boundaries that a family develops between itself and the outside world. These internal/external boundaries allow information and contact to flow to and from the family.

If these boundaries are flexible, the family is open to new information and experiences. This kind of "open system" allows the family to evolve and adjust to life cycle changes more easily by discarding unworkable or obsolete interactive patterns. If the family has a "closed system," it tends to be "insular" and "not open to what is happening around it." These families can even be "suspicious of the outside world" (Goldenberg and Goldenberg 2005, 375). Families which tend toward closed systems boundaries have much more trouble with the process goals of adapting to the many changes families must learn to navigate.

If Mrs. Dutta were to see a family therapist, the therapist would listen to Mrs. Dutta's story from this systems perspective. The therapist would quickly make several connections between Mrs. Dutta's symptoms and her family situation. The therapist would see Mrs. Dutta as the identified patient but not as the source of the problems. Instead, the therapist would understand the locus of difficulty to be at the level of the family itself. The family therapist would see Mrs. Dutta's family as having difficulty processing the life-cycle change of Mrs. Dutta coming to the United States. The prior equilibrium that the family had achieved was disrupted by this event and the family has not been able to rebalance itself.

The family therapist would see vulnerabilities in the family which likely contributed to this difficulty. The first is that the family has fairly rigid inside/outside boundaries which leaves it relatively enmeshed and isolated from contact and communication with the outside world. There is almost no place in the story where the family unit connects with others outside itself, except in the highly proscribed roles of school and work. In addition, the spousal subsystem of Sagar and Shyamoli seems to be weak or at least insufficiently strong to withstand Mrs. Dutta's arrival. The tensions between Sagar and Shyamoli are overwhelming the bonds between them and these tensions are not being dealt with directly. Mrs. Dutta has become the scapegoat for their problems.

Plus, there are signs that a triangulation is occurring as Shyamoli feels that Sagar's loyalty has shifted to his mother. From Shyamoli's perspective, Sagar does not support her in the marriage and sets no limits on Mrs. Dutta. Shyamoli has a litany of complains with Mrs. Dutta—she throws away perfectly good food, leaves dishes dripping all over the countertops, orders the children around, cooks whatever and whenever she likes, takes over the entire kitchen, and leaves the house and all of their clothes smelling like grease (Divakaruni 1999, 45).[1] It has gotten so bad that Shyamoli feels like "this isn't even my house anymore" (45). And, yet, she gets no support from Sagar. As Shyamoli explains, "You're too busy being the perfect son, tiptoeing around her feelings. But how about mine? Aren't I a person too?" (45) All Sagar can say in response is "Hush, Molli, the children . . ." which Shyamoli quickly reminds him are already deeply aware and intertwined in the problems (45). Without help, the family is unable to process these issues and Mrs. Dutta is stuck bearing their burden.

Indeed, it would be particularly striking to the family therapist how closely Mrs. Dutta's symptoms are tied to the family's problems. After all, it was just after the tensions erupted into an open confrontation between Shyamoli and Sagar that Mrs. Dutta's symptoms took their most severe turn. When Mrs. Dutta hears that the bond between her son and daughter-in-law has become so tenuous that Shyamoli is threatening to leave, Mrs. Dutta falls into the darkest depths of her depression and retreats to her room in cold despair (46). The connection between Mrs. Dutta's symptoms and her family's dysfunctions would make it clear to the family therapist that Mrs. Dutta does not have an individual problem. Mrs. Dutta's symptoms are a direct result of these many family difficulties.

Based on this assessment, the family therapist would recommend family sessions to help the family work through these problems. The therapist would help the family reframe Mrs. Dutta's problem so that they better understood her symptoms as emerging from larger family relations. The therapist would help them see that treating Mrs. Dutta alone would likely result in a return of symptoms if the family context were not addressed. The therapist would explain that a typical course of family therapy runs from 10 to 20 sessions depending on how things go. She would ask to see the entire family at first and would engage with the family by "accommodating to their transactional style as well as assimilating their language patterns and manner of affective expression" (Goldenberg and Goldenberg 2005, 389). The therapist would help each member feel supported and safe to give voice to previously unexpressed feelings and problems. By "joining" with the family in this way, the therapist would let Mrs. Dutta's family "know they are understood and cared about, and that in such a safe climate they can begin to confront divisive family issues" (2005, 389).

To facilitate change, the therapist would adopt an active, problem-solving approach that would challenge rigid, repetitive family patterns.

The therapist would strive for a balance that is "supportive and nurturing at some points and challenging and demanding at others" and that moves "swiftly in and out of emotional involvements without losing track of family interactions and transactional patterns" (2005, 397). Once a supportive alliance was set up, the therapist would use family "enactments," or role-playing techniques, to bring family struggles into the session. The therapist would encourage the family to act out their dysfunctional transactions rather than just talk about them. The immediacy of this technique would allow the therapist to directly observe the process instead of relying on family recollections and reports. The therapist could then "intervene on the spot and witness the results of such interventions as they occur" (2005, 392). The therapist might also use a "family sculpting" technique which would asks family members to take turns as family "director" placing "each of the other members of the family in physical space" (2005, 392). This technique reveals individual perceptions of "family boundaries, alliances, roles, subsystems and so on" (2005, 392). Through these techniques, the therapist would help "unfreeze" the family's repetitive patterns and guide them to modify their interactions.

The family therapist would work to open the family boundaries so that it becomes less enmeshed and more open to outside contact and communications. Plus, she would be particularly attentive to spousal subsystem problems. She would schedule some conjoint sessions with Sagar and Shymoli to help them work through their interpersonal difficulties. From the story, it is clear that Sagar and Shymoli are struggling with conflicts over Mrs. Dutta and that they have ineffective communication patterns. Other problems that often show up in family are conflicts over money, over power and control, and sexual incompatibilities. By meeting with Sagar and Shymoli as a couple, she will be able to address these problems more deeply and she will reinforce the integrity of the spousal subunit.

The narrative outcome of family therapy for Mrs. Dutta would be that she would come to understand her sadness in relation to broader tensions in the family. Through the course of family work both she and the family would develop "more effective coping skills and learn better ways to ask for what they want from one another" (2005, 399). They would take steps to loosen their internal/external boundaries and therefore create a more open family system. With increased contact and input with others— including perhaps other families from the Indian diaspora—they would gain more support and more perspective for their problems. Plus, the family would be able to resolve many of their unworkable patterns, to adopt new rules and realignments, and to achieve "more flexible family interactions" (2005, 393). Even if they were unable to do these things, they would recognize that these family problems are important and they would have learned problem-solving techniques for addressing new or remaining issues together. The family therapist would also continue to be available to the family. As Mrs. Dutta's family makes progress, the sessions would be spread out from weekly, to biweekly, and eventually to every three months. After a year or so, Mrs. Dutta's family may officially terminate from the therapy, but the therapist would be available for additional sessions as needed years into the future—whenever the family gets stuck in a dysfunctional sequence. The narrative outcome for the family would be that they now understand these are signs that the family needs assistance.

Humanistic Psychotherapy

As discussed in Chapter 3, humanistic psychotherapy emphasizes four central themes:

1. A phenomenological approach that views the client as the expert of his or her own experience.
2. A deep commitment to human capacities for self growth and actualization.
3. A belief in the human agency as the final arbitrator of choice and self-determination.
4. A person-centered focus that includes a deep respect for the uniqueness of each individual. (Rice and Greenberg 1992, 198–99)

Different humanistic therapies work with these themes in different ways. Of the three leading alternatives—person-centered, Gestalt, and existential—the most influential (at least in the United States) is Carl Rogers's person-centered approach.

Rogers began his psychotherapeutic work by applying a traditional diagnostic, prescriptive, and professionally impersonal stance. But his experience with clients left him so disenchanted with this approach that he switched tactics. Indeed, he practically reversed his previous stance. He "tried listening and following the clients lead rather than assuming the role of the expert" (Raskin and Rogers 2005, 135). Over time, he drew on a phenomenological analysis of people's experience to develop a form of therapy that put understanding the person's subjective experience at the heart of the therapeutic enterprise. Rogers aimed to mirror the client's phenomenology as faithfully as possible, without disagreeing, contradicting, or giving insight from the therapist's perspective. The goal was to create an environment of trust and understanding from which the person could develop his or her own solutions and stimulate his or her inborn capacity for growth and development.

The open and candid self-exploration Rogers aimed for could be achieved only in the context of a close and trusting relationship. Rogers carefully articulated what he came to see as the three most essential ingredients of this kind of helping relationship: congruence, empathy, and positive regard.

Congruence refers to the therapist's ability to be present and transparent to the client. The therapist works with the client without facade and does not pretend to be something he or she does not feel. If negative feelings emerge, such as boredom or perhaps a transient dislike, the therapist shares these experiences with the client. This "does not mean that the therapist blurts out impulsively any attitudes that come to mind. It does mean, however, that the therapist does not deny to himself or herself the feelings being experienced and that the therapist is willing to express and be open about any persistent feelings that exist in the relationship" (2005, 146). Within the boundaries of the therapeutic relationship, the therapist therefore provides the client with a genuine relationship rather than what could be called a "pseudorelationship" that gives in to the temptation to hide behind a mask of professionalism.

Empathy focuses on the importance of understanding the client's perspective from within the client's frame or reference. As Rogers put it, empathy is "an active experiencing with the client of the feelings to which [the client] gives expression, the counselor makes a maximum effort to get under the skin of the person with whom he is communicating, he tries to get within and live the attitudes expressed instead of observing them, to catch every nuance of their changing nature; in a word, to absorb himself completely in the attitudes of the other" (2005, 145). The therapist refrains from imposing upon the client his or her own interpretations or perspectives. Instead, the therapist works to mirror the client as faithfully as possible; he or she does not disagree with the client, point out contradictions, or suggest that the client is defensive or unaware of deeper-level meanings. To be empathic, there is "simply no room for any other type of counselor activity or attitude; if he is attempting to live the attitudes of the other, he cannot be diagnosing them, he cannot be thinking of making the process go faster" (2005, 145).

Positive regard is the third essential ingredient for person-centered therapy. Other terms that have been used for this ingredient are warmth, acceptance, nonpossessive caring, and prizing. Positive regard involves the therapist's nonjudgmental accepting attitude toward the client as a contextual whole that allows the client to feel whatever he or she may feel at the moment. "It involves the therapist's willingness for the client to *be* whatever immediate feeling is going on—confusion, resentment, fear, anger, courage, love or pride" (2005, 145). Rogers refers to positive regard as a "kind of love," comparing the notion of "love" to the theologian's term *agape,* which "respects the other person as a separate individual and does not possess him. It is a kind of liking which has strength, and which is not demanding" (quoted in Shaffer 1978, 84).

Central to Rogers and other humanistic psychologists is the metaphor of a person as an "organismic self." In stark contrast to the mechanistic models of self found in biopsychiatry of cognitive behavioral approaches, this organismic self is present at birth, has inherent strivings of its own, and, most important, has an inborn capacity for self-repair and self-actualization (1978, 81). Rogers found that the three therapeutic ingredients mentioned above allowed this inborn capacity, or organismic self, to regenerate. When the therapeutic conditions were met—when Rogers was able to be real, deeply accepting, and empathically in tune—the people he worked with rediscovered a capacity for growth. These conditions were the soil, the sunlight, and the moisture needed for healthy growth and regeneration. When people were supplied with these conditions, they were able to work out within themselves an understanding of the aspects of their life causing pain or dissatisfaction. They reorganized their personality and their relationships with life in ways that were more rewarding and fulfilling. They showed fewer "neurotic" or "psychotic" symptoms and more characteristics of healthy, well-functioning people. In addition, clients came to value themselves more highly, were more confident and self-directing, and were more open to experience and more accepting of others.

Rogers argued that "whether one calls it a growth tendency, a drive toward self-actualization, or a forward-moving directional tendency, it is the mainspring of life, and is, in the last analysis, the tendency upon which all psychotherapy depends. It is the urge which is evident in all organic and human life—to expand, extend, become autonomous, develop, and mature." For Rogers, the task of therapy was to revitalize the person's natural healing capacity. People's tendency toward growth "may become deeply buried under layer after layer of incrusted psychological defenses; it may be hidden behind elaborate facades which deny its existence; but it is my belief that it exists in every individual, and awaits only the proper conditions to be released and expressed" (Rogers 1961, 35).

With this background in mind, what would a person-centered therapy look like for Mrs. Dutta? Person-centered therapy is similar to other therapies in that the therapist would be available for meetings with Mrs. Dutta to help her work through her difficulties. The difference would be in the therapist's style. Rather than approach Mrs. Dutta as an "expert" who "knows" the causes of her mental suffering (as would happen with a biopsychiatrist, a psychoanalyst, or a cognitive therapist), a person-centered therapist would work toward creating a therapeutic relationship in which Mrs. Dutta could develop her own understandings and resolutions to her troubles. The humanistic therapist would work to reinvigorate her natural healing capacity rather than try to fix "broken brains" or "cognitive distortions."

To get a sense of what this approach might look like, it helps to look closely at the relationship Mrs. Dutta has throughout the story with Mrs. Basu. Interestingly, Mrs. Dutta uses her relationship with Mrs. Basu to set up a form of person-centered therapy that is similar to what Rogers would recommend. Mrs. Dutta's self-created person-centered therapy takes the form of an internal dialogue she has with Mrs. Basu as she writes her a letter.

In this internal dialogue, Mrs. Dutta finds a conversational partner who is everything Rogers describes. Mrs. Basu is congruent and deeply empathic and has unconditional positive regard. The "therapy" with Mrs. Basu begins when Mrs. Basu uses her letter to pose a simple and open-ended question: "Are you happy in America?" Because Mrs. Basu is not present in the story (except in Mrs. Dutta's mind), this turns out to be the only question Mrs. Basu asks. Yet the question seems to work to stimulate the process of person-centered therapy. Mrs. Dutta realizes that if she is to answer Mrs. Basu she must be honest and real about it. She has known Mrs. Basu for too long for her to give superficial answers or for Mrs. Basu to be "fobbed off with descriptions of Fisherman's Wharf and the Golden Gate Bridge" (31).

As Mrs. Dutta works through her feelings about being in the United States, the imaginary Mrs. Basu listens with deep empathy. Mrs. Basu does not try to correct or contradict Mrs. Dutta when she admits how much she misses her life back in Calcutta or that she finds her grandchildren to be a disappointment (33). Even when Mrs. Dutta tries to give a glib presentation of herself in the United States—"I'm fitting in so well here, you'd never guess I came only two months back. I've found new ways of doing things, of solving problems creatively. You would be most proud if you saw me"—Mrs. Basu seems to understand this sentiment without judgment.

Finally, throughout her internal dialogue with Mrs. Basu there is a warm sense of positive regard for Mrs. Dutta. Mrs. Basu is Mrs. Dutta's "closest friend," whom she has known for more than forty-five years going back to the time she was first married (31). Although friendship as we normally think of it (with reciprocal and parallel obligations and interactions) is not a requirement of person-centered therapy, Rogers does use the term *agape* (ancient Greek for nonsexual love or friendship) to capture what he means by the "positive regard" that the therapist must feel for the client. It seems clear throughout the story that Mrs. Basu has this kind of "deep liking" for Mrs. Dutta that Rogers has in mind. The affection that Mrs. Basu feels is also unconditional and unpossessive. Mrs. Basu has such a long relationship with Mrs. Dutta that she sees her as a whole and does not judge her for any one thing she might do or say. She values her at an overarching level that is independent of moment to moment events.

It must be said that the internal dialogue that Mrs. Dutta has with her imaginary Mrs. Basu is different from one she would have likely had with the actual Mrs. Basu (using "actually" loosely considering this is fiction). When Mrs. Dutta was preparing to leave Calcutta, the actual conversations Mrs. Dutta had with Mrs. Basu were hardly an ideal person-centered exchange. They were the opposite. Mrs. Basu contradicted Mrs. Dutta on her plans to give away her tea set, "Have you gone crazy?" (38), and she directly confronts Mrs. Dutta on her plan to sell her house, "What if you don't like it there [in America]?" (39). When Mrs. Dutta tries to explain her reasons, Mrs. Basu responds with a skeptical and seemingly critical "I wonder" (39).

But none of this is present in Mrs. Dutta's imaginary conversation with Mrs. Basu. Instead, Mrs. Basu seems to understand and to appreciate only Mrs. Dutta's feelings. And, most of all, she seems to feel a "real liking" for Mrs. Dutta as she goes through her troubles. In this way, the imaginary Mrs. Basu works for Mrs. Dutta like a person-centered therapist would work. These conversations provide Mrs. Dutta with the necessary ingredients to figure out her own problems. And, just as Rogers predicts, the relationship is instrumental in helping Mrs. Dutta find new resolutions to her troubles, get unstuck from her current situation, and restart her own processes of growth and development.

Conclusion

The three models reviewed in this chapter—interpersonal, family, and humanistic—provide compelling ways to understand Mrs. Dutta's troubles. But they do so by focusing on very different variables than the previous models I discussed. Interpersonal and family models move away from the more individualistic concerns of the last chapter. For interpersonal and family models, Mrs. Dutta is a subset of a larger system, and the most important variables are not "inside" Mrs. Dutta but in her relations with friends and family. Humanistic approaches turn the wheel again to focus on existential/phenomenological variables of experience, free will, and personal growth. Carl Rogers provides an understanding of Mrs. Dutta that is much less "pathological" than the other models reviewed so far. For Rogers, Mrs. Dutta is going through a healing process. All she needs to recover spontaneously is the warmth and nurturance of an empathic, kindly, and sympathetic companion.

Each of these models can clearly be applied to Mrs. Dutta. As in the last chapter, if Mrs. Dutta were to work with a therapist using one of these models, she would gain the narrative tools needed to make sense of her troubles, to move forward in her life, and to weave the story of her sadness into her ongoing narrative identity. But, once again, we cannot stop here. Even though the six models reviewed thus far cover the range of therapies most common in the clinical community, there remain a host of other models that might be invaluable for Mrs. Dutta.

CHAPTER EIGHT

Alternative Stories

SPIRITUAL THERAPY, EXPRESSIVE THERAPY, AND CULTURAL, POLITICAL, AND FEMINIST THERAPIES

MAINSTREAM CLINICAL STORIES only begin to help us imagine alternatives for Mrs. Dutta. This means that narrative psychiatry must look to additional clinical stories for important narrative resources. There are a host of additional approaches on the margins of what we could call "clinical" and many more that move beyond the clinics all together. As a group, I refer to these additional possibilities as "alternative stories," and the ones I address include spiritual therapy, expressive therapy, and cultural, political, and feminist therapies.

Spiritual Therapy

Religious and spiritual approaches to psychic difference come from three broad sources: transpersonal psychology, "New Age" alternatives, and specific religious traditions. There are overlaps in these domains, but they all form separate narrative communities, so it helps to review them separately rather than lump them together. Transpersonal psychology initially emerged as a branch of humanistic psychology. Like humanistic psychologists, transpersonal psychologists go beyond the limits (as they see them) of psychoanalysis and cognitive behavioral psychology to explore the full breadth of human meaning and experience. Transpersonal psychologists go even further than most humanist psychologists, however, and have become known as a "fourth force" in psychology because of their willingness to explore the transcendent dimensions of human consciousness—the so-called transpersonal or spiritual dimensions.

These transcendent experiences are difficult to describe and must be considered ultimately enigmatic. Nevertheless, efforts at articulation can be helpful for understanding and evoking these states. Transpersonal psychologist Ronald Valle attempts to "word" the unwordable by describing six characteristics common to transpersonal experiences. These include (1) a feeling of stillness and peace along with a deep sense of being or "isness" that exists behind all thoughts, emotions, and sensations; (2) an all-pervading aura of love and contentment with all that exists; (3) a feeling of connection to a larger whole that diminishes and dissolves the notion of an individual ego; (4) a radical forgetfulness of the body boundaries and a feeling infinite space; (5) a sense of time hovering or standing still and merging together into an ultimate eternal now; and, finally, (6) bursts or flashes of insight that have an "other-than-me" quality about them, as if the thoughts and words that emerge independently from the person are a manifestation of something greater and/or more powerful than the self alone (Valle 1989, 259).

These states of consciousness resemble experiences of mystics from multiple religious traditions throughout the ages. Thus transpersonal psychologists are deeply interested in what Aldous Huxley once called "perennial philosophy" (Huxley 1945). They often turn their attention to wisdom from spiritual traditions such as Hindusim, Yoga, Zen, Buddhism, Taoism, Christian mysticism, Judaism, and Native American cultures. Transpersonal psychologists are generally less interested in becoming devotees to these practices and more in using these traditions for spiritual insights useful for therapeutic guidance in a more secular world.

A similar willingness to learn from Eastern religious traditions for spiritual guidance also characterizes a wealth of "New Age" approaches to psychotherapy. There are too many of these approaches to review in detail, so I will focus on two options that provide particularly insightful metaphors for depression. These come from New Age healers who use Yoga and those who use meditation in the care of sadness. Yoga techniques for depression are worked out in great detail by Amy Weintraub in her book *Yoga for Depression*. Weintraub first became interested in depression through her own experiences. She was treated with mainstream psychotherapy and medication with little response; so she turned to Yoga for help. Within a year of Yoga practice, she felt much better and was no longer taking medication. She was so impressed with the power of Yoga breathing and posture techniques along with the wisdom of the Yogi tradition, she decided to become a certified Yoga teacher.

Weintraub uses Kripalu Yoga practices that provide a systematic method for maintaining physical and emotional health. Kripalu Yoga teaches that sadness and suffering come when we are too tightly bound to current reality and therefore cut off from the greater cosmos. "As we live farther and farther from the truth of our wholeness, we become ignorant of that wholeness and live as though we are separate and alone" (Weintraub 2004,13). Yoga practice provides an opportunity to wake up from ignorance, "to transcend our identification with our bodies, our clinging to what we love, our avoidance of what we hate, our fear of death" (2004, 13). Ultimately, practicing Yoga leads to a "healing state, a blissful feeling wherein you may lose the sense of yourself as a being separate from the universe and gain a momentary sense of union" (2004, 12).

A similar New Age alternative for depression evolves from the traditions of Zen meditation. Philip Martin's book *The Zen Path through Depression* provides a good example. Like Weintraub, Martin turned to New Age therapeutic practice as a result of own experiences. At the age of thirty-seven, he went through a devastating depression despite the fact that he had been practicing Zen Buddhism for many years. He first approached his sadness from a mainstream perspective and saw it as a "disease" completely separate from his spirituality. Martin felt his depression was not only separate from his spirituality but also the opposite of his spirituality. Depression stole all he found life-giving including his spiritual practice. He therefore felt that his religious and spiritual life had little to offer him in this darkest hour. Spirituality was about transcendence, but Martin felt his depression was pulling him down more than elevating him. "If there is one thing depression is not about it is transcendence. It is instead an experience of being stuck in the mud, unable to rise up through the muck like the lotus flour so often used as a metaphor in spiritual teaching" (Martin 1999, xii).

But separating his depression from his spirituality turned out to be a passing phase. With time and continued devotion Martin found a way to connect his sadness and despair to his Zen practices. Ultimately, he discovered that the downward movement of depression allowed him to settle more fully into his spiritual life and provided an opportunity for spiritual opening and learning. Depression, Martin concluded, "is not just of the body and mind, but also of the heart. Depression offers us an opportunity to deepen our spirit, our lives, and our hearts. There is much that we can learn about ourselves and our world through this journey. Through attentive compassionate practice with depression, it is possible to experience an even deeper healing, and grow in our spiritual lives" (1999, xii).

Martin went on to become a psychiatric social worker and a workshop leader so he could share his experiences with others. His book provides a guide to the wilderness of depression through a series of meditative practices loosely based on Zen and Buddhist teachings. Martin shows his readers how to sit in a quiet place either in a lotus position or on a cushion or chair with their hands folded in their lap and their gaze dropped a few feet in front of them. He explains that it helps to sit upright with one's spine comfortably settled and with one's chin tucked in slightly. The meditator then allows his or her attention to move from the head, through the neck, shoulders, and chest, and to settle in the belly. Once the person is comfortable, Martin suggests the following:

> Feel the rising and falling in your of your belly as you breathe in and out. If you wish, you may think "in" and "out" with your breathing.
>
> Become aware of the space around you. Feel that this is your space, your ground, your home. You are like a pebble sinking down through a river to settle on the bottom, where the waves and currents can't touch you. Envision yourself sitting on a throne, or a mountaintop—anywhere that seems a powerful place to you. Say three times to yourself, "this is where I make my stand." You are immoveable here. You are strong and safe in this spot. All fears, all grief, all pain can come and wash over and through you, and not wash you away.
>
> Now come back again to your breath, following it in and out, as your belly rises and falls. Your breath is the anchor that is always there, that will hold you in this place. Become aware that this place where you sit is immense and extends into all directions. It is large enough to contain whatever you choose to invite in. Welcome your feelings of fear, your pain, your depression into this place. Tell the depression that it need not feel excluded from this place, that in this place it will receive understanding and compassion. Invite into this place as well any deities, energies, that you wish. Especially those that give your strength—but also, if you would like those that may

bring your fear. Again come back to your breath, and feel the immensity of the place within which you sit like a mountain.

When you are ready to return, remind all those you have invited in that they are welcome to return again when you come back. Remind yourself that this place waits for you, at any time you wish it. Sit, enjoying this place your have created. Let your attention rise through your chest, shoulders, and neck, and slowly open your eyes. (1999, 5)

Martin gives guided meditations like this for many of the most difficult aspects of depression: pain, fear, doubt, anger, suffering, loneliness, death, desire, and impermanence, among others. He shows how to ease these feelings through meditations and how doing so may enrich the soul while it mends the spirit. Stopping and listening to depression through meditative practices calls the meditator to the most profound questions of living: Why are we born? Why must we suffer and die? Who are we? How shall we live in this moment? These questions, along with the pain and suffering that accompany them, are the seeds of freedom. Painful and frightening as this approach to depression may be, the rewards can be immense. When the person who has depression takes a stand and does not run, he or she learns what depression has to teach. "To do so is not to give in to depression, but rather to take the first step in healing our pain and suffering" (1999, 3).

Cheri Huber, a teacher of Zen meditation, takes a similar approach to depression but goes one step further. Although Martin teaches how it is possible to welcome depression into one's meditative space, he does so with the intent of changing or working through the depression. This idea—the idea that depression should be changed—is an idea that runs through all the approaches we have reviewed so far. For Huber, in contrast, the idea that one must change depression can be one of depression's most painful dimensions. Rather than try to change their sad and painful feelings, Huber suggests that Zen meditative practices allow people with depression to accept themselves at a deeper level and to embrace themselves with love and compassion. This embrace does not happen after the depression passes but "RIGHT NOW!" (Huber 1999, 1). If you are depressed, you should be depressed. "This moment is the only moment you have. HAVE IT! Don't be afraid to experience your experience. There is nothing to fear. . . . Nothing awful is going on except the way [you] feel, and if [you] didn't hate the feeling, it wouldn't be awful" (1999, 107–8).

How we treat ourselves in depression, in other words, may be more important than getting over depression. "Hating or rejecting this moment is not good practice for loving and accepting myself in another" (1999, 108). Huber therefore uses meditative practices to help people to feel what they feel and think what they think. "Whatever you are doing, love yourself for doing it. Whatever you are thinking, love yourself for thinking it" (1999, 133). And, most important, even if you don't like the feelings of sadness or despair, "love yourself for not liking it" (1999, 133).

Outside transpersonal psychology and New Age alternatives like Yoga and meditation, attention to the spiritual dimensions of psychic life occurs within specific religious traditions. In these traditions, transcendent experiences are less the exception and more the ordinary outcome of religious life. Practitioners of a religious faith regularly consider their spiritual life to be an important aspect of their overall well-being. The most common metaphorical structure for understanding and organizing the relationship between religious life, psychic difference, and psychic pain is the notion of a "dark night of the soul." Spiritual directors often meet people who are going through periods of intense psychic pain with feelings of emptiness, meaninglessness, loneliness, depression, and despair. These intense states, or "dark nights" as they are often called, tend to occur in two periods of a devotee's life: (1) during incubation periods just before a spiritual breakthrough into a new, different, and ultimately higher level of spiritual practice or awareness, or (2) during times when a devotee has gotten too far away from his or her religious practice.

The first of these "dark nights" resembles what William James famously called the "twice-born." For James, the heart of religious experience comes precisely from its capacity to transform melancholy feelings of meaninglessness, ominous evil, and deep personal guilt. Religion, for James, is explicitly understandable as an invaluable response to these most dire of human states. When people go through a religious conversion, they break through to the other side of these dark feelings. They become "twice-born," and they achieve a state of assurance and salvation. Meaningfulness emerges, there is a triumph of ultimate goodness, the world becomes more beautiful and real, and there is a "loss of all worry" with a "sense that all is intimately well with one." The twice-born have feelings of peace, harmony, and a "*willingness to be*, even though the outer conditions remain the same" (James 1982, 248). In addition, the twice-born are empowered to the point that previous inhibitions and conflicts often melt away (Taylor 2002, 37). James calls this alternative psychic state "saintliness," which brings the direct feeling of a greater power and a corresponding sense of elation and freedom. In saintliness, "the outlines of confining selfhood melt down," and there is a "shifting of the emotional center towards loving and harmonious affections" (James 1982, 271–73).

The second form of "dark night" is similar except that it occurs not at a moment of spiritual breakthrough but at times when a person gets too distant from his or her religious roots. For this form of dark night, Agenta Schreurs uses the evocative phrase "spirituality in exile" (Schreurs 2002, 45). The phrase refers to a spiritual practitioner who has wandered, or who has been forced, too far from his or her spiritual homeland: someone who has lost his or her sense of belonging and is left isolated and alone. Schreurs finds that spirituality in exile is particularly common in contemporary Western cultures because the lure of a material and secular life distracts people from their religious practice. The religious devotee who has lost touch with his or her religion often goes through the melancholic pain of spiritual exile that includes all the painful emotions James describes. These feelings are not a sign of pathology for religious practitioners but a potent signal that guides the devotee back to the fold of religious faith and tradition.

Using this overview of spiritual approaches as a guide, we can see that if Mrs. Dutta were to approach her sadness and despair from a spiritual direction, there would be a range of therapeutic options available for her. She could work with a transpersonal psychotherapist, she could get involved with a variety of New Age spiritual practices such as Yoga or meditation, or she could develop a renewed commitment to her Hindu religious traditions. There is little in Mrs. Dutta's story to suggest how she might react to either a transpersonal or a New Age therapy. However, scholars of Indian diaspora do find that Indian women to be open to a range of alternative approaches to emotional troubles, and it is possible that Mrs. Dutta would fit this pattern (Guzder and Krishna 2005, 125). If so, Mrs. Dutta might get considerable relief from working in transpersonal therapy or through New Age options.

Although it is plausible that Mrs. Dutta could gravitate toward a transpersonal or New Age approach, instead of speculating on these possibilities I will stay close to the story and focus the rest of my spirituality discussion for Mrs. Dutta on the directly religious option. It is possible that Mrs. Dutta would be more attracted to religious approaches than secular approaches. Indian psychotherapist Kushalata Jayakar explains that "even though most Indians have been readily absorbed into the mainstream of American workforce, the majority have remained unchanged in their basic spiritual beliefs" (Jayakar 1994, 166). Thus these beliefs continue to have a major influence on many Indian women's view of the world and their place in it.

Jayakar argues that key features of Hindu belief systems include the importance of dharma and karma. *Dharma* may be defined as "the traditional established order, including all individual, moral, social, and religious duties" (1994, 166). Every person has his or her own personal dharma, which is largely determined by contextual factors such as "stage in the life cycle, particular hierarchical relationships, caste, and individual temperament" (1994, 166). *Karma* may be defined as deeds or emotions that contribute to life as a "continuous cycle of birth, death, rebirth, and death" (1994, 167). Many Hindus believe that "one's destiny is to repeat this cycle indefinitely unless one performs deeds that allow one to be reborn in a higher form" (1994, 167). If a person gives in to the emotions of lust, anger, greed, want, and envy to perform evil deeds, the result will be rebirth in a lower form. Conversely, if a person gives up material and worldly attachments, "the cycle of karma is broken and one enters the stage of *Nirvana* or *Moksha*" (1994, 167).

The belief structures of dharma and karma mean that for practicing Hindus their emotional life, interpersonal life, and spiritual life are all interconnected. When Hindu practitioners use religion to find peace at the emotional and interpersonal level, they make not only emotional and interpersonal progress but also spiritual progress. In addition, they may well achieve access to ineffable transcendent experiences described by William James and the transpersonal psychologists. As a result, many South Asian women turn to "religious and spiritual practices to deal with personal distress, often with positive results" (Guzder and Krishna, 2005, 126).

Certainly for Mrs. Dutta there is considerable evidence in the story that she continues to be highly influenced by her religious beliefs. While she was a young bride and was having great difficulty coping with her new husband's family, she would pray every night "to Goddess Durga, please let me sleep late, just one morning!" (Divakaruni 1999, 30).[1] And even now, as she tries to cope with her son's family in America, she often lays in bed in the morning reciting "the 108 holy names of God. *Om Kesavaya Nama, Om Narayanaya Namah, Om Madhavaya Namah*" (31).

Throughout the story we see also Mrs. Dutta drifting away from her previous spiritual practices now that she is living in America. Cut off from her previous community, she longs for her "Thursday night Bhagavad Gita class" that she used to attend with her friend Mrs. Basu (39). In addition, Mrs. Dutta has to give up any notion she had of passing her spiritual traditions to her grandchildren. Anticipating the possibility of providing spiritual guidance for the children, Mrs. Dutta brought them a "vellum-bound *Ramayana for Young Readers*" with the hopes of sharing it (35). But the children only push the book away somewhere to the back of the closet. And, worst of all, when Mrs. Dutta asks her grandchildren to sit with her while she chants her evening prayers, they respond only with impatience and the "most transparent excuses" to return to the television or to talk on the phone with their school friends (35).

Thus, the narrative seeds are present for Mrs. Dutta to understand her current sadness and despair as a kind of "spirituality in exile." She could use this insight to make a renewed commitment to her faith and her religious practices. Either she could do this in America, or it could be part of an explanation for returning to Calcutta. Either way, Mrs. Dutta's return to her faith could be the process through which she not only moves through her despair toward self-contentment but also achieves an even a higher level of spiritual peace and transcendence.

Expressive Therapy

The key metaphorical structures for expressive therapy parallel those of the creative process, and thus expressive therapy draws out similar features between the therapeutic work and creativity. For the expressive therapist, both the artist and the person in therapy have in common the need to explore their internal psychic life and their relations to the surrounding world. Both the artist and the person in therapy use this awareness to transform their experiences through self-expression. Building on this metaphor, expressive therapists focus their attention along a continuum that places more or less emphasis on the therapy side or on the artist side, so that one side of the continuum may be called "art *in* therapy" and the other side "art *as* therapy" (Edwards 2004, 1). The distinction sounds subtle, but the lived experience between these two approaches can be tremendous.

The expressive therapist working from the art *in* therapy side of the continuum uses artistic expression to help the person access psychic materials that can then be processed through a therapeutic relationship. Art *in* therapy therefore functions similar to the way Freud used free association and dream analysis. Artistic expression helps the person and the therapist tune into aspects of the person's thoughts, feelings, and perceptions that are difficult for the person to reach through direct conversation alone. Once this material becomes available through art, expressive therapists help the person process the material and work it through in ways similar to those used by other therapists.

At the other end of the continuum, when the focus is on art *as* therapy, the expressive therapist focuses less on standard therapeutic goals and more on helping people achieve creative expression. This side of the continuum makes sense because art alone, independent of traditionally defined therapeutic goals, can be tremendously healing for several reasons. First, many people find art to be deeply engaging. When a person is absorbed in the process of art, other aspects of life, even painful aspects, may drift into the background. Plus, art allows people to take hard-to-reach experiences and share them with an audience. These experiences, which might otherwise be toxic or alienating, find a voice through creative expression so that the artist is no longer isolated and alone with them. In addition, art rewards people for their sensitivity. To be an artist, one must be able to pick up on aspects of inner life and the world that often escape other people. This sensitivity, which is often coded negatively in the context of most therapies (most therapeutic approaches suggest that people "stop being so sensitive"), is coded positively in the context of creative expression. A highly sensitive "patient" may be a bad thing, but an highly sensitive "artist" is nearly always a good thing. Finally, art takes experience that may otherwise be seen as ugly or inappropriate and turns it into something aesthetically beautiful or politically moving (or both). Art therefore brings the artist outside his or her own preoccupations and into the community. It gives people an invaluable role in making the world a better place.

Expressive therapists vary in how much they emphasize art *in* therapy compared with art *as* therapy. Some primarily focus on the former, some on the latter. Most focus on a combination. It is important to note, however, that the farther we move toward the art *as* therapy side, the more the therapeutic language recedes and the creative language emerges. If one goes far enough down this continuum, artistic work easily escapes the context of expressive therapy altogether and becomes simply art. In other words, one does not need to be in expressive therapy to do artistic work. One may simply become an artist. The practical implications of becoming an artist will mean not going to a therapist at all but rather taking art classes, setting up a studio, joining an artistic community, and the like. The ideas and language of "therapy" may be the farthest thing from the artist's mind.

If we apply expressive therapy models to Mrs. Dutta, we can imagine a future for her in which artistic work becomes an important part of her therapeutic process. Of the many expressive modalities Mrs. Dutta might pursue, writing seems to be the one that connects most closely to what we know about her. It is even fair to say that Mrs. Dutta's biggest preoccupation throughout the story is not her troubles but her writing. After all, the story is titled "Mrs. Dutta Writes a Letter." The letter Mrs. Dutta writes in the story is meant for Mrs. Basu, but if Mrs. Dutta were to build on this writing interest, a range of possible futures could open for her. She might generalize from her specific writing preoccupation to writing more broadly, and this could be further developed in the service of therapy, the service of becoming a writer, or in some combination the two.

In the popular Indian magazine *Life Positive*, Ritu Khanna provides a lovely window into how Mrs. Dutta might get involved in writing therapy. Khanna's article, "The Write Spirit," begins by exploring the question of how the writing process can be therapeutic. She describes some of the positive effects of writing she finds: "Writing is a meditation: it settles the mind. It is a de-stressor: it releases tension. It is like a confessor who keeps your secrets safe. It is also a mood-changer, with the capability of making you happy. It is an outlet, for it helps you let go of your negative thoughts. It is creative, cathartic, curative. Quite simply, writing is beyond words" (Khanna 1996). Khanna goes on to make the point that writing can be therapeutic for everybody—not just for people who write professionally. In the article, she interviews several people of all ages who have found writing invaluably therapeutic. "Sakshi Kapur, 10, ties the key to her diary around a friendship band securely arranged around her wrist. Reeti Desai, 12, is inspired by Anne Frank. Meena Gupta, 47, begins to write two months after her 13-year-old son's death and finds strength in words. Nimmi Kumar, 58, takes an oath to write the name of Sai Ram and an artist is born. Vijai Shanker, 62, uses it to express himself" (1996).

Khanna discusses several writing genres, but one that comes up repeatedly is journal writing. She quotes Indian neuropsychiatrist Avdesh Sharma, who recommends that patients keep a "stress diary" that records daily stressors and their effects. The stress diary is not just an occasional activity but a long-term commitment and a skill to be cultivated. The process of writing journal entries on specific problems give diarists time to reflect, problem-solve, vent feelings, and see patterns in their lives. In this way, serious and systematic journal writing functions in a way that is similar to psychotherapy. It "gives direction to your life, but, most important of all, it gives you a sense of control over your thoughts" (1996). Journal writers use their journaling to get in touch with themselves, to discover practical solutions to life difficulties, and to uncover suppressed issues that might otherwise remain frightening and painful.

Depending on circumstances and her inclinations, Mrs. Dutta could easily follow the suggestions of Khanna to pursue journal writing for her sadness. Or she could go even further with her writing interest. Rather than use journal writing primarily in the service of therapeutic goals, she could decide that she would like to pursue writing classes with the goal of becoming a writer. Creative writing instructor and accomplished author Carolyn See provides a good example of how creative writing can be therapeutic even without traditional therapeutic goals. We can use See's book, *Making a Literary Life: Advice for Writers and Other Dreamers*, to illustrate the kind of instruction Mrs. Dutta might receive were she to sign up for writing classes (See 2002). See describes her instruction as meant for beginners and outsiders, people who are "timid, forlorn and clueless," and for "students just coming to the discipline, older people who wanted to write in their youth and never got around to it, [or] folks who live in parts of the country where the idea of writing is about as strange as crossbreeding a tomato and a trout" (2002, xi). In other words, See teaches writing for people much like Mrs. Dutta.

See emphasizes that the first step in developing a writing life is self-exploration. She suggests that in times of quiet reflection writers pay attention to their thoughts, their feelings, and their perspectives on the world around them. She advises people: "Listen. What's your 'voice,' what's your material, what's your genre, what are you trying to say?" (2002, 10). See gives the example of how she first developed her own voice. Interestingly, it first happened in a psychotherapy session. See was recounting to her therapist a long and painful exposé of the worthless doings of her husband. Her emotions began to rise, her volume became louder and louder, and eventually she shouted to her therapist, "I can't stand it!! I can't *stand* it!" (2002, 10). Her therapist listened quietly and responded calmly: "Oh, you seem to be standing it all right" (2002, 10). This simple remark was an epiphany for See. She realized in a flash that there was another way to be with her "suffering." Her intense feelings were not destroying her as she imagined, and she was "standing them all right." See realized that she need not try to remove these feelings. Instead, she could use them in her art. She could make them her writing material and the core of "her voice."

Through listening to herself rant (what better way, after all, to find "your voice" than by listening to yourself), See discovered that she was "Queen of the long sentence. Much given to exaggeration and embellishment. *Addicted to italics.* Empress of the long held grudge" (2002, 10). This voice was one thing when it existed solely in the context of complaining about her life but something entirely different when transformed into art.

> "So, you know what he did *then*? There he was, in the home of his
> girlfriend, and his shirt was hung right there over the doorknob—
> I always wondered what happened to that shirt—and there she is
> sitting on her little couch sobbing, and he's in a chair, falling over
> laughing, and I'm sobbing along with her and I'm saying, 'All right,
> Tom, you have to choose between us *right now*,' but he's laughing so
> hard he can't even get the words out. . . ."
> "So what did you do then?"
> "I guess I just went home. Because I had to take care of the baby."
> (Voice rises again.) "Because she had that terrible *fever*! A hundred

and five degrees! And he's out fucking his *brains* out with the dreaded Jennifer." (2002, 10–11)

See makes it clear that she would not have picked this voice for her art, or this material for that matter, if she had her first choice. She would rather have the voice of her favorite authors, like the "measured, morally right voice of E. M. Forster" (2002, 11). But it was not to be. There was no point trying to fake it. Her own voice pushed up—"insistent as steam from a teakettle"—and it made much more sense to develop it than to deny it.

For See, the wonderful thing about becoming a writer is that it opens a "crystal door in your mind" (2002, 15). When you are trapped in painful situations, like sorrowful memories, an unpleasant argument, or listening to a droning bore, being an artist allows you to "turn pain into pleasure." What was once merely painful experiences now becomes valuable material. "Wake up! Keep waking up! Wake up more and more often. Look at your life with the 'keen, trained eyes of the novelist' " (2002, 15). By paying attention to your life in this way you can gradually develop "your voice, your characters, your world view, your genre of choice. When you've thought about this, discreetly, for weeks or days or years, you can start—silently!—to write" (2002, 17).

We can imagine that if Mrs. Dutta stayed with writing classes like the one See would teach, she might end up with a writing voice similar to that of Chitra Divakaruni, the author of "Mrs. Dutta Writes a Letter." Like Mrs. Dutta, Divakaruni was born in India and lived in Calcutta before immigrating to the United States. Unlike Mrs. Dutta, Divakaruni came to the United States when she was a young woman and while she was here received a Ph.D. in English from UC Berkeley. Because Divakaruni now teaches writing, it is even possible to imagine Mrs. Dutta taking a class from Divakaruni. If so, she might have an experience not unlike that of Lisa Pamphilion, a returning student, who took one of Divakaruni's classes: "At first I felt really old, but Dr. Divakaruni made me feel okay because she's really down to earth and she's got a sense of humor, . . . I looked at her as a role model and a mentor" (Softky 1997, 27). Whoever Mrs. Dutta's teacher might be, it is easy to imagine her and Divakaruni developing similar voices. Divakaruni's work is partially autobiographical, most of her stories set in the Bay Area of California, and she often deals with immigrant women's experience. In addition, Divakaruni's writing tends to unite people by breaking down stereotypes and dissolving boundaries between people of different backgrounds, communities, and ages. As she puts it, "Women in particular respond to my work because I'm writing about them, women in love, in difficulties, women in relationships. I want people to relate to my characters, to feel their joy and pain, because it will be harder to [be] prejudiced when they meet them in real life" (quoted in Softky 1997, 27).

Mrs. Dutta could develop a similar voice in her writing. She would not need to have the same worldly success as Chitra Divakaruni to be successful as a writer. Mrs. Dutta might write for friends, family, classmates, and smaller presses, journals, and blogs. Whether she was read widely or locally, she might still enjoy the same sense of pride and purpose that Divakaruni surely must feel in her own work. As Carolyn See puts it, through consistent work, play, and luck writers can achieve "enough publication, reputation, and recognition to make [them] happy" (See 2002, xii). Not only that, they can most certainly achieve a "literary life" that in itself is an invaluable achievement. When people develop a literary life, their artistic practice helps them avoid butting their head futilely against the many frustrations and disappointments of daily life. As See explains, this can happen "wherever you are, wherever you live, and whoever your family and friends may be" (2002, xii).

Cultural, Political, and Feminist Therapy

Cultural, political, and feminist approaches to psychic pain and difference all use the metaphorical structure of a social model that moves beyond individual metaphors to consider the larger sociocultural context of the individual's situation. In this way, social models are similar to family models and interpersonal models except that social models consider cultural and political dynamics outside the scope of these other models. Tyrer and Steinberg point to four basic tenets of the social model:

1. difficulties are often triggered by life events outside the individual,
2. social and cultural forces linked to status and role often precipitate difficulties,
3. mental disorders often become and remain "disordered" because of societal influences, and

4. much apparent mental disorder has been falsely labeled and should be regarded as a temporary maladjustment. (Tyrer and Steinberg 2005, 100)

The most mainstream use of social models comes under the label "cultural competence." Culturally competent therapy requires the therapist to develop three cultural capacities: cultural awareness, cultural knowledge, and cultural skill. *Cultural awareness* involves a deep sensitivity to the phenomenon of culture and the often invisible sets of rules, norms, values, expectations, and rituals that form the cultural matrix of all human life. This awareness also includes an appreciation of the way that cross-cultural exchanges often involve multiple forms of ethnocentric devaluing of the "other." *Cultural knowledge* goes beyond a basic awareness of the phenomenon of culture to develop a deep familiarity with particular cultures and subcultures. To fully appreciate cultural influences on individual lives, one must not only be aware of the phenomena of culture but also know the person's particular cultural background in a multifaceted way. One must know that culture's particular history, customs, founding figures, ways of life, definitions of the good, and so on. Finally, the clinician must have the *cultural skill* to bring cultural awareness and cultural knowledge into the clinical encounter so that the variables of culture can be properly included in understanding people's problems and in helping them consider options (Campinha-Bacote 1994).

Cultural competence approaches usually do not develop whole new models of therapy but encourage all clinicians to develop cultural capacity. Peter Tyrer, a British professor of community psychiatry, went further than most when he developed the skill set of cultural competence to the point of introducing a new model of therapy he calls "nidotherapy." The term "nido" comes from the Latin word *nidus*, or nest. Tyrer argues that a bird's nest is an ideal metaphor for understanding human cultural embeddedness. Using this metaphor as a guide, a nidotherapist will look to see whether a person's presenting difficulties have more to do with his or her cultural location, his or her "nest," than with the particular person. "The aim is to help the individual take up an acceptable role again, not to correct a biochemical disturbance, exorcize an unresolved conflict or recondition behavior. In many instances it will be realized quickly that the person being seen for help is not really unwell at all and is just in the wrong place at the wrong time" (Tyrer and Steinberg 2005, 110). Nido-therapy makes no attempt to change the person or the larger culture but rather works with the person find the cultural environment in which he or she best fits. Tyrer finds that "once the changes are made, the state of patient-hood is no more" (2005, 111).

Cultural competence, including more robust versions like nidotherapy, focuses on cultural difference more than cultural politics. A more radical and political use of social models shows up in a group of theorists and therapists who became collectively labeled "antipsychiatry." Authors in this group, such as Erving Goffman (1961), R. D. Laing (1967), Thomas Scheff (1999), and Thomas Szasz (1974), differed widely in their philosophies, but their main tenet was clear. "Mental illness" is not an objective medical reality. Instead, either the term "mental illness" is a negative label used for social control, or what we call mental illness is a political strategy for coping in a mad world. As Laing put it, "the apparent irrationality of the single 'psychotic' individual" may often be understood "within the context of the family." And the irrationality of the family can be understood if it is placed "within the context of yet larger organizations and institutions" (Laing 1968, 15). Put in social context in this way, psychic pain and difference have a political legitimacy of their own that is often erased by models of psychic difference that emphasize pathology. Rather than a pathology, mental difference and suffering can be the beginning of a personal and social resistance or of a healing process and should not be suppressed through therapeutic interventions.

Feminist models of therapy build on a social model, and they have arguably done the most to integrate both cultural and political forces in their work. Feminist therapists strive for a continuous political examination of their own personal values, a consistency between their feminist perspectives and their therapy work, and a deep understanding of the roles that both cultural difference and cultural politics (such as the politics of gender, race, economic status, sexual orientation, ageism, ableism, and other axes of denigration and subordination) play in women's and men's lives. As a result, the integration of feminist approaches into therapy becomes more than an add-on; it becomes "a complete transformation in the way in which therapy is understood and practiced" (Enns 2004, 9).

Feminist therapies center around the key metaphor for all of feminist work: *the personal is political.* Carol Hanisch first coined this phrase in the early years of second-wave feminism when she noted how feminist political discussions tended to get mired in debates over personal verses political priorities (Humm 1992, 1). Hanisch's experience in early consciousness-raising groups made it clear that these debates rested on a false binary: "One of the first things we discover in these groups is that personal problems are political problems." Hanisch found that intimate personal conversations with other women gave her a "political understanding which all my reading, all my 'political discussions,' all my 'political action,' all my four-odd years in the movement never gave me. I've been forced to take off the rose-colored glasses and face the awful truth about how grim my life really is as a woman" (Hanisch 1971, 152–53). Hanisch argued persuasively that the two issues—personal and political—are much intertwined, and her phrase "the personal is political" became a rallying cry not only for feminist psychotherapy but also for second-wave feminism more broadly.

Using this model as a guide, feminist therapists see many of the problems people bring to therapy not as individual pathology but as the consequences of oppression and signs of internalized oppression. Dana Crowley Jack provides a good example of this approach with regard to depression in her book *Silencing the Self: Women and Depression*. Early in her career, Jack was struck with the fact that the rates of depression are twice as high for women as for men, and she set herself the task of understanding what it is about "women's inner and outer worlds that creates this vulnerability to the hopelessness and pain of depression" (Jack 1991, 2). She found herself deeply dissatisfied with mainstream psychoanalytic and cognitive approaches that failed to address gender. The major concepts used in these approaches—attachment, loss, dependence, self-esteem—too often organize people's problems through a hidden lens of patriarchal values and norms. She argued that the masculine/paternal preferences for self-sufficiency and independence embedded in nonfeminist models are far from neutral: "Ego strength has come to be equated with lack of reliance on others for emotional support; self-reliance is seen as mature and reliance on others as immature" (1991, 6). As a result, feminine/maternal preferences for relationships and emotional intimacy come to be pathologized as neurotic and dependent. "A woman is caught in a double bind: society still pushes her to define herself through [feminine/maternal] relationships, but then it invalidates her wish for connection by derogating the importance of attachments" (1991, 6).

When Jack considered women's vulnerability for depression through this perspective, she found that feminine/maternal women often complained of "losing themselves" when they were in relationships with masculine partners. One of her clients, Susan, put it this way: "I like closeness. I like companionship. I like somebody, an intimate closeness, even with a best friend. I was always so close to my mother. . . . I was used to that all through my childhood, having an intimate closeness . . . someone that shared my feelings, my fears, my doubts, my happiness, my achievements, my failures. And I've never had that with my husband. I can't talk to him on those levels. . . . He lives in a very concrete, day-to-day, black-and-white world" (1991, 4). Susan, like many others, came to see her needs for closeness as a sign of dependence and weakness. She had the feeling that her "need for intimacy" and "deep level of friendship or relationships with people was sort of bad," and she began to believe "there was something the matter" with her (1991, 5).

Jack observes that Susan uses the language of patriarchy to deny what, on another level, she values and desires. Further, the patriarchal power dynamics of her relationship with her husband forces her to stifle these desires. "Susan cannot ask for what she wants most—an intimate closeness. Hidden from her description is the reason why she cannot ask: inequality mutes her ability to communicate directly about her needs. She does not feel entitled to have her needs filled, nor does she feel they are legitimate" (1991, 5). Susan is forced to bury part of her self to relate to her husband, and over time this self-silencing combined with a sense of inferiority leads to feelings of despair, hopelessness, and worthlessness. From Jack's perspective, these depressed feelings arise not from individual pathology; instead they are the expectable outcome of oppressive environments and the internalization of oppressive values.

For women of color, the gender dynamic Jack describes are often further complicated by ethnopolitical issues. Lillian Comas-Diaz points out that women of color exposed to dominant Western white cultures often experience what could be called "cultural Stockholm syndrome" or "postcolonization stress" disorder (Comas-Diaz 2000, 1320). Racism and cultural imperialism impose dominant values as inevitable and superior, leading minority groups to accept not only dominant cultural values but also the prevailing negative stereotypes of their own group. This internalized colonization can create pervasive feelings of identity conflict, alienation, and self-denial that can further lead to psychological effects of shame, rage, and depression. "Consequently, the experiences of racism, sexism, identity, conflict, oppression, cultural adaptation, environmental stressors, plus internalized colonization prevalent amount and specific to many women of color, constitute critical considerations in the delivery of relevant psychotherapeutic services" (Comas-Diaz 1994, 288).

Because feminist therapies have done the most to integrate social model insights into their therapeutic efforts, I will use feminist therapy as my prototype for this section. If Mrs. Dutta saw a feminist therapist, the therapist would put the many cultural and political dynamics of Mrs. Dutta's situation at the forefront of their work together. Mrs. Dutta's feminist therapist would quickly tune in to the deep struggle Mrs. Dutta is having adjusting to her new cultural environment. Mrs. Dutta struggles with the isolation of her new suburban life and misses the crowded living and the street life of Calucutta (40). She feels adrift in the strange customs of the United States, embarrassed by the casual exposure of underwear (36), confused by the idea of "invaded privacy" (40), and insulted by the odd holiday of Mother's Day: "Did the sahibs not honor their mothers the rest of the year?" (34). She cannot fathom the scandalous amounts of television her new family watches every night. This nightly television ritual not only takes away time that Mrs. Dutta would like to use talking and connecting but also leaves her alienated, as she is unable to understand the jokes or to make sense of the television worlds that absorb her family (29–30).

Mrs. Dutta feels particularly estranged by the food customs of her new home. Although she tries to provide the family with proper Indian foods, like "puffed-up chapatis, fish curry in mustard sauce, and real pulao with raisins and cashews and ghee," the family prefers to eat low-fat foods or things that are quick, like Rice-a-Roni or frozen burritos (33). In addition, Mrs. Dutta finds cross-generational relations to be out of sync with what she knows. The children are allowed to close their doors at night against their parents, leaving the parents unable to enter their rooms without knocking (31). And when the children complain that Mrs. Dutta takes up too much time in the bathroom, she expects them to be severely punished for such a display of disrespect (32). Instead, the children are indulged to the point that Mrs. Dutta finds her head pounding with "anger at the children for their rudeness" and with their parents for "letting them go unrebuked" (32). The total effect is that, if she is honest with herself, Mrs. Dutta's grandchildren leave her with a "heaviness [that] pulls at her entire body" when she thinks of how they are a "disappointment" to her (33). She feels the children are hopelessly lost in a world of American values, to the point of developing American voices consumed with a glittering world of "Power Rangers, Metallica, and Spirit Week at school" (35).

Listening through the metaphor of "the personal is political," Mrs. Dutta's feminist therapist would also pick up the many gender, race, and postcolonial dynamics of her situation. With regard to gender, Mrs. Dutta's story makes it clear that she has lived her entire life within a strict patriarchal order. In Calcutta, as a young wife, she was forced to wake up before her husband's family to make them all breakfast despite her desperate wish to sleep late. If breakfast was not right on time, she was harshly scolded by her mother-in-law until she was left in tears (29). Mrs. Dutta coped with this situation by internalizing the patriarchal edict (just as her mother-in-law before her had done): women are supposed to be "*good wives and daughters-in-law, good mothers. Dutiful, uncomplaining. Never putting ourselves first*" (43; italics in original). If women get out of role, they should be punished (44). Mrs. Dutta is accordingly flummoxed by her daughter-in-law's American notions of more equal relations between the genders. She cannot accept, for example, the idea that her son would be asked to do the laundry: "No, no, no, clothes and all is no work for the man of the house" (37). Nor can she get used to the idea that "here in America we don't believe in men's work and women's work" (37). Just because her daughter-in-law works outside the home, as does her son, there is no reason from Mrs. Dutta's perspective that she should not also continue her wifely duties.

The political dynamics of race and nation status are also prevalent in Mrs. Dutta's story. Mrs. Dutta's feminist therapist would note that Mrs. Dutta's family, as a whole, could be said to have "postcolonization stress disorder." They have all been required to accommodate themselves to the norms of a dominant, colonizing culture that has demanded the sacrifice and eradication of their cultures of origin. Mrs. Dutta's son, daughter-in-law, and grandchildren are all trying to live a fully assimilated American life with little left of their Indian heritage. This might seem like simply a choice they have made, but the powerfully felt hidden forces of racism and colonization weighing down on them and insisting that they pass became all too apparent in the encounter Shyamoli, Mrs. Dutta's daughter-in-law, has with her neighbor. Mrs. Dutta made the cultural mistake of hanging out laundry in the wrong place, and the neighbor rebuked Shyamoli for the event: "Kindly tell the old lady not to hang her clothes on the fence into my yard" (45). The rebuke, though it may have seemed benign, left the otherwise confident Shyamoli shaking and raw with pain: "She said it twice, like I didn't understand English, like I was a savage. All these years I've been so careful not to give these Americans a chance to say something like this, and now . . ." (45). In this incident, the feminist therapist would see years of racial and postcolonial pressure on the family to become culturally white and Western if they hope to fit in.

Mrs. Dutta's feminist therapist would use this assessment of the cultural, gender, and political conflicts of her life and her current situation to begin helping Mrs. Dutta work toward solutions. The therapist would be clear that Mrs. Dutta's depression is not a personal problem but a cultural and a political problem. The solution, therefore, would have less to do with individual change and more to do with cultural and political change (Brown 1994, 38). Perhaps, like in nidotherapy, the therapist and Mrs. Dutta would work together around the possibility that Mrs. Dutta return home to Calcutta. Depending on Mrs. Dutta's interest or willingness to engage in the politics of her situation, returning home could be seen as merely a "better fit," or it could be seen as a political statement and intervention. If Mrs. Dutta felt open to engaging in political struggle, she could use feminist therapy to see her move to Calcutta as a resistance against the notion that the "West is best." She could also see the move as forming solidarity with other women in India. Mrs. Dutta's decision to move in with her friend Roma and drink tea together while fighting off gossip and backlash could be seen as a more than personal solution. It could be the beginning of a larger political plan to help women in India who find themselves oppressed by role stereotypes.

And moving to India would not be the only option that might arise from feminist therapy. Mrs. Dutta might, for example, find a similar solution without returning to Calcutta. She could stay in the United States and find an Indian cultural community where she could connect with other women going through similar problems. If she was so inclined, she could engage in cultural politics with these women around the many tensions surrounding Indian women's diaspora.

It is important to emphasize that for feminist therapist the goal will not necessarily be complete removal of personal distress. If personal distress is a sign of political tension, removal of distress is not necessarily a good thing. After all, the distress not only signals a political problem but also provides motivation for political change. Laura Brown provides a good example of how continued stress may be a positive outcome in therapy. She describes a client who started therapy depressed and how, after therapy, the client's depression was not completely gone. Instead, it morphed in a new direction. After therapy, the client's depression "no longer disempowers her or serves as a source of isolation" (1994, 38). The pain became less about the client herself and was no longer debilitating or confusing. "Rather, she is distressed—angry and outraged—by . . . social and political realities that were formerly obscured from her view by the teachings of patriarchy and finely by her own wounds from that same system. Her anger fuels her social activism—her writing, speaking, and teaching about the political realities that she has uncovered in her healing process" (1994, 39). In short, the client remains depressed, but the meaning of the depression changed.

Conclusion

These alternative ways to narrate sadness, like the mainstream options reviewed in the last two chapters, provide important resources for narrative psychiatrists. Though alternative approaches are not in the mainstream, they continue to have tremendous narrative value. Alternative models are every bit as effective as mainstream approaches for helping an imaginary Mrs. Dutta develop a new narrative identity—an identity that could transform her sadness or her relationship to this sadness.

In the next chapter, I pull back from the details of these last three chapters and return to the question of how a narrative psychiatrist would operate in view of his or her deep awareness of Mrs. Dutta's many options. In addition, I consider the relation of narrative psychiatry to recent work in bioethics and recovery-oriented psychiatric care.

CHAPTER NINE

Doing Narrative Psychiatry

H OW CAN PRACTICING clinicians make sense of the last three chapters? For many psychiatrists there will be something deeply disquieting and disorienting about the exercise. Many psychiatrists will have internalized their training in science, data, and clinical trials and will be distant from the worlds of literature, narrative, and theories of meaning. Seeing Mrs. Dutta's story interpreted in vastly different ways can go against the grain of this clinical training because the hidden pedagogy of science contains an unstated ontology of *one, and only one, true world*. Clinicians identified within this ontology will find it hard to make sense of the possibility that all these interpretations of Mrs. Dutta could be "true." After all, there's only one Mrs. Dutta. There must be only one truth of her situation. For these psychiatrists, the idea that all these interpretations could be "true" borders on the absurd, even the insane.

And yet the evidence in our interpretive exercise puts the seeming absurdity of multiple interpretations in question. The work we did in the last three chapters shows that "Mrs. Dutta Writes a Letter," like so much of literature, lends itself easily to different and multiple interpretations. Divakaruni did not write the story as an exercise for mental health workers. She was surely not even thinking about the many different clinical and alternative meanings to Mrs. Dutta's sadness. Yet what is most fascinating about our interpretive exercise is that each new interpretation was easily relevant to Mrs. Dutta's situation and few of the interpretations had to stretch. If Mrs. Dutta came to see a psychiatrist at the time of her crisis, or worse, if she came after her darkest despair had continued for a few weeks, she would easily receive a diagnosis of major depression. However, there are still multiple ways Mrs. Dutta could proceed. The story contains seeds of a biological interpretation but also a psychoanalytic one. It contains kernels for a cognitive behavioral therapy but no more so than for family therapy. It opens itself to a humanistic reading but also a political, spiritual, and creative reading, just to name a few. Each new approach foregrounds aspects of the story that were left out by the previous approach. Each allows us to make sense of Mrs. Dutta's troubles, each provides metaphors for selecting key elements of attention, and each provides guidance for the future. Each could be used by Mrs. Dutta to help restory her troubles, and each provides the fundamental plot structure of a new narrative identity.

It is critical to have a firm sense of this phenomenon before doing narrative psychiatry because this is exactly the background awareness needed for narrative work. The practical implication of this awareness is that a narrative psychiatrist would have a deep appreciation of the multiple options available for Mrs. Dutta. With this awareness in mind, if Mrs. Dutta came to see a narrative psychiatrist, the first step would be to use the tools of narrative medicine to develop an empathic connection with Mrs. Dutta. This step helps Mrs. Dutta move beyond her isolation with her situation, and, as discussed earlier, this step alone can be one of the most healing tools that clinicians can offer.

The next step would be to help Mrs. Dutta make choices about how to proceed. Following the basic ethical principle of informed consent, the narrative psychiatrist would give Mrs. Dutta background on the array of treatment options so she could make informed choices. The narrative psychiatrist would explain that she herself practices a narrative approach that integrates resources from a variety of treatment models and beyond. This approach recognizes that any number of therapeutic schools can be helpful for people and that a variety of insights and strategies can be woven together to form a hybrid narrative of a person's past, present, and future that can be helpful. The issue of medication would be included in the mix of therapeutic options. The narrative psychiatrist would explain that many psychiatrists would recommend medication treatments either alone or in combination with psychotherapy for severe depression. The narrative psychiatrist would explain the risks and benefits of the medication options along with a careful review of the outcome studies for the medicine's effectiveness. The decision of medication, like decisions about other options, would remain with Mrs. Dutta.[1]

If a narrative and integrative approach like this were to sound good to Mrs. Dutta, she and the narrative psychiatrist would continue working together. If not, the psychiatrist would work with Mrs. Dutta to find a suitable referral. If they do continue working together, whatever Mrs. Dutta decides with regard to medication, the larger frame of narrative psychiatry stays intact. With or without medications, the goals for the clinician and Mrs. Dutta will be to develop an empathic understanding of her lived experience, form a good-quality therapeutic alliance, and find acceptable resolutions for her troubles. At the time of Mrs. Dutta's crisis and when we imagine her coming to therapy, she seems to have run out of possibilities. Her story seems to have led to a dead end, and her feelings of hopelessness and helplessness seem like her only options. What possible hope for a satisfactory resolution can there be in the face of such despair?

This is where the past one hundred years of clinical literature along with the thousands of years of broader cultural wisdom can be extremely helpful. Taking the larger view of the possible options, medication treatment can be seen as a small part of this broader clinical and cultural wisdom. With or without medication, in all likelihood, there is something in the long history of working through human problems that could be helpful for Mrs. Dutta.

From a narrative perspective, therefore, a major therapeutic task for Mrs. Dutta and her therapist will be the task of curiosity. The therapist and Mrs. Dutta will need to be curious about the kinds of resolutions people have thought of in the past and use this curiosity to explore these options together. The fruits of this curiosity will be to see whether any of these previously developed options, or some combination of options, will provide hope and possibility for Mrs. Dutta. As Louis Pasteur once put it, chance favors prepared minds. Flashes of imagination and creative insight do not just happen in a vacuum; they are the product of preparation. In Mrs. Dutta's situation, the chance that the narrative clinician and Mrs. Dutta will find a resolution that fits Mrs. Dutta's values depends on how well they have prepared their mind—how much they know about possible options and how creative and successful they can be at applying those resolutions, or some combination of them, to Mrs. Dutta's situation.

Both Mrs. Dutta and her narrative clinician will bring a great deal of preparation to the task. They both have heard thousands of stories over the course of their lifetime about how people resolve crisis and how people evolve beyond being stuck in bad situations. The clinician, as a narrative clinician, will have attended a lifetime of plays and films and will have read widely in the world of fiction, memoir, and biography all with an eye to their relevance for clinical work. In addition, the narrative clinician will have attended closely to the wisdom of clinical literature and the data of clinical research for insights on how Mrs. Dutta could proceed.

Mrs. Dutta's "case" highlights how narrative psychiatry can easily blend research data and outcome studies with a larger narrative frame. Narrative psychiatry recognizes that research data can be helpful in decision making, but, unlike more typical evidence-based medicine (EBM) approaches, narrative psychiatry pays equal attention to the question of patient values. In this way narrative psychiatry works well with what philosophical psychiatrist Bill Fulford calls "values-based medicine" (VBM). The first principle of VBM gets to the heart of the issue: "All [clinical] decisions stand on two feet, on values as well as on facts, including decisions about diagnosis (the 'two feet' principle)" (Fulford 2004, 208). This means that data alone cannot determine clinical decisions and choices of diagnostic models. Even in cases where there are good data to support a clinical diagnosis and intervention, that alone does not determine the decision. The final decision still depends on how the intervention lines up with the person's life choices and life goals.

Fulford gives an example of an artist who ultimately decides against taking lithium even though there were good data to support its use (and even though it helped her calm her hyperactivity) because the experience of lithium reduced her capacity to visualize color. For the artist in Fulford's example, the effect of lithium on her experience of color was more important than its effects on her moods. The artist preferred to "diagnose" and intervene in her problems through a creative/expressive model rather than a biomedical one. Data alone could not determine this decision.

Similarly, in the context of informed choice, whether or not Mrs. Dutta opted for medication, the narrative psychiatrist would be perfectly comfortable with her decision (including her decision to change her mind at a later date). Narrative psychiatry, in other words, does not denigrate biological explanations, disease models, or psychopharmacologic treatments for mental states. However, and this is critical, narrative psychiatry also does not idealize disease models of explanation and treatment. For the narrative psychiatrist, medication questions involve not only biological effects and side effects but also the effects and side effects of organizing one's psychic life through a biomedical frame. Some people will choose, or not choose, this frame independent of the details of particular medications.

For narrative psychiatry this makes perfect sense because biological explanations are not an exception to the narrative psychiatry's general understanding of the ways that metaphor and plot work to shape narrative identity. Medical models function as metaphors, and like other metaphors they create a kind of "seeing as." It is true that when people inhabit scientific frames they come to experience "seeing as" in a deeply naturalized way, to the point where "seeing as" becomes "being as" ("I have a chemical imbalance"). But this process is not different from other uses of metaphor to structure experience—it is just another example of the role of metaphor and linguistic structures in the formation of narrative identifications. Once one enters a metanarrative perspective, the option of a biomedical model becomes a choice, just as a humanistic model or a cognitive behavioral model would be.

In addition, this common ground between psychological and medical treatments opens up to the issue of common therapeutic factors, sometimes called "placebo effects," in medication treatments. It is well known that much of the effectiveness of medications, as with psychological treatments, comes from the therapeutic alliance (Greenberg 1999). The presence of these common-factor aspects of medication treatment provides a key advantage to narrative approaches to using medication. Narrative psychiatrists put empathic connection in the foreground of their work, which means that their clients have an excellent chance of developing quality therapeutic alliance. And this alliance will account for a major portion of the therapeutic effect regardless of the specific tools used—including the tool of medication.

There are many ways this could play out with Mrs. Dutta. She may come to the narrative psychiatrist with clear-cut ideas about how she would like to go forward. She may say, "I don't want to spend a lot of time whining about this stuff, I want you to give me some medication to make it go away." Or she may say, "I am not a medication person, and I won't take medication. I want to find other ways to deal with this problem." Or she might say, "I saw a TV show about how helpful cognitive therapy can be for depression, I would really like to give that a try." Or it could be that Mrs. Dutta does not have an advance preference. She might say something like, "I have no idea how to proceed. You're the doctor—what would you suggest?"

In any of these situations, the early work would be to help Mrs. Dutta gain a fuller sense of her options. If she already comes with a preference, the narrative psychiatrist would offer to situate her preferences within the context of other options. If she does not have a preference, the narrative psychiatrist would outline the most common alternatives. Included in both of these presentations would be the option of a narrative integrative approach that remains open to the many options and their possible combinations. It would be clear in this presentation that the choice of approach rests with Mrs. Dutta. Part of this process would be deciding whether Mrs. Dutta and the narrative psychiatrist should work together. If the approach Mrs. Dutta wishes to pursue is one that the narrative psychiatrist is competent to provide, that would certainly be an option.

The expected outcome would be that if Mrs. Dutta engaged with a particular model, or if she worked with a narrative psychiatrist who helped her weave together a new hybrid option tailored to her sensibility, she would create a correlating story that would connect with her sadness. This new story would become an important strand in the tapestry of stories that makes up her sense of self. It would organize her understanding of how her past contributed to her present sadness, and it would organize her future relationship with that sadness. Mrs. Dutta's new narrative identity would provide a new way of being with her sadness with new goals, new interpersonal relations, and new rituals. When a new way of being is developed, Mrs. Dutta's sense of sadness would be transformed and reconfigured. If this did not happen, Mrs. Dutta and the narrative psychiatrist would have the option of trying harder or longer or changing approaches.

To make sense of this flexibility of approach and outcome, it helps for practicing clinicians to rethink the hidden pedagogy of their clinical training. This means rethinking how a clinical science background has trained us to think in terms of *one, and only one, true world*. Much of the challenge of this rethinking has to do with the meaning of the term *world* in that phrase. Philosopher Clive Cazeaux provides a helpful analysis of the term and shows the metaphorical role it played in the much discussed science wars of the 1990s (Cazeaux 2007, 139). The science wars involved a heated dispute concerning the question of whether science *discovers the world* or whether science *constructs the world*. Both sides of the science wars appealed to the "world," but each used a different metaphor to understand it. Defenders of science as discovery understood it in terms of an ultimate reality independent of human cognition. Defenders of science as construction understood it in terms of phenomenology of experience—something much more akin to the idea of a worldview or zeitgeist. The same term, *world,* brought up very different associations for the competing sides, and the metaphorical oscillation between world as ultimate reality and world as zeitgeist created the either/or conditions of a bitter science wars battle without compromise.

Many clinicians, steeped in a clinical science background, adopt the ultimate reality metaphor for "world," and this puts them on the discovery side of the science wars. But clinicians do not have stay true to their training, nor do they have an obligation to enlist in the science wars. They can put their background in perspective by recognizing the metaphorical nature of what they have been taught. In addition, they can avoid the science wars all together by adopting new metaphor for "world" beyond the oscillating options of it as ultimate reality or as zeitgeist. If clinicians adopt an understanding of "world" that combines these two meanings, as a *narrative perspective on ultimate reality*, they can avoid science wars fighting all together.

This combined narrative perspective on the notion of "world" allows clinicians to understand that the conflicting interpretations of Mrs. Dutta are alternative takes on ultimate reality, alternative points of view. None of these competing perspectives "discover" the final reality of Mrs. Dutta's situation, nor do they completely "construct" her situation. Each provides a narrative perspective that evokes, highlights, and foregrounds some aspect of her real situation while simultaneously backgrounding other aspects. By rising above their clinical training to adopt a new metaphor for "world" outside the dueling possibilities of the science wars, clinicians can embrace the possibility of multiple perspectival realities of Mrs. Dutta's situation without it seeming absurd or insane.

Narrative psychiatry provides the tools for practicing clinicians to reach this possibility, and the evidence of the Mrs. Dutta exercise suggests that narrative affords multiple advantages for clinical practice. By adopting the narrative approach of multiple worldviews, practicing clinicians avoid not only the science wars but also the tired debates in the clinical world between antipsychiatry and propsychiatry. Narrative approaches allow clinicians to interpret Mrs. Dutta's story without denigrating any single worldview (by calling it a "myth") and simultaneously without idealizing any one view (by calling it the "objective truth" or ultimate reality). And finally, narrative approaches do this without falling into "anything goes"–style relativism. The approaches people choose matter greatly. Indeed, the approaches people take shape their identity and their future. Which narrative people choose not only organizes the past and present but also provides a compass for going forward. Even though the stakes are high, the options are still many. There is no one path that people must pursue. Adopting this kind of flexibility and sophisticated narrative nuance creates practicing clinicians who avoid dogmatism—the bellicose insistence on any necessary "one way"—and who are open to helping clients find the path that best suits their needs and desires.

This is why narrative psychiatry works well as a theoretical scaffold for therapeutic model integration. Narrative integration allows clinicians to put the client's needs, desires, and model preferences above the clinician's allegiance to any particular training or school.[2] It signals a clinician's willingness to learn from and potentially apply a range of different approaches. In this way, narrative integration contains much of the needed humility that Dr. Chekhov so effectively articulates. It is true that many psychiatrists already practice a form of spontaneous narrative integration through the commonsense wisdom they have gained in clinical practice. But, unfortunately, spontaneous integrative approaches are easily attacked by holders of single models, or a cocksure version of combination models, as being muddled or confused. This attack can make it seem that a clinical willingness to take seriously the varieties of psychic life is somehow a weakness or a fault. And, worse yet, clinical integrationists can often internalize this critique and feel insecure and even inferior about their practice.

Narrative theory is immensely helpful here because it argues that metanarrative clinical integration can be a rigorous position and that a willingness to be open to multiple models is not less desirable than a single-model approach. Narrative clinical integration is not necessarily better—no point in getting dogmatic about it—because the question of "better" always depends on particular goals and desires. But, generally speaking, narrative integration is just as good as single-model approaches. And, depending on the goals and desires of the clinical encounter, narrative integration can be better.

Bioethics and Recovery: Two Important Trends Pushing toward Narrative Psychiatry

As the preceding discussion highlights, narrative psychiatrists make a much needed move away from a paternalistic, "doctor knows best" approach to clinical care. It is important to understand that the call for this move away from paternalism and toward increasing consumer empowerment is bigger than narrative psychiatry. Outside narrative psychiatry, two powerful forces are also pushing psychiatry toward greater consumer empowerment—the bioethics movement and the recovery movement. Both call for a reform of psychiatric practice toward more consumer-directed care. Only by adopting the skills and tools of narrative can psychiatry meet the reform imperatives of these movements.

The major consequence of the bioethics movement through the 1960s and 1970s has been the shifting of clinical care from a beneficence-centered model to an autonomy-centered model. In a beneficence-centered model, the highest value for the clinician is to do good for the patient based on the clinician's judgment about the patient's needs. This model, at its extreme, can become deeply paternalistic. In contrast, in an autonomy-centered model, the highest value for the clinician is to respect the person's wishes and informed choices about his or her body and life. How clients should be treated depends, in short, on their goals and desires—not the clinician's goals and desires. In an autonomy-centered model the value of beneficence does not vanish. Doing well for patients remains a goal, but when that goal conflicts with the patient's wishes, beneficence has to take a back seat in favor of the patient's wishes. As I outlined in Chapter 2, the bioethics movement set the stage for narrative medicine. Once patient autonomy became a priority in medical encounters, it became imperative that clinicians have the tools to empathically connect with their patients. Otherwise, how would they even know patients' desires and goals? Psychiatric ethics has been less influential than medical ethics, but it is only a matter of time until the bioethics movement affects psychiatry as well. When it does, it will stimulate a more narrative approach, just as it did in medicine.

In addition, the past thirty years have brought the rise of a consumer movement in psychiatry that similarly works to transition clinical encounters away from paternalistic, expert-knows-best value structures. Recently this consumer movement has blossomed from a marginalized subgroup of ex-patients to a deeply robust "recovery movement" that remains controversial in psychiatry but has flourished in community psychiatry settings (Sowers and Thompson 2007). A major force driving the recovery movement is the increasing chorus of criticism against psychiatric insistence on what are seen as one-dimensional medical model approaches. This chorus of criticism comes from consumer activists, critical mental health providers, and interdisciplinary academics working at the interface of psychiatry, disability studies, and cultural theory (Bracken and Thomas 2005; Double 2006; Lewis 2006a, 2006b; Morrison 2005; Tamini and Cohen 2008). Interestingly, like the earlier deinstitutionalization movement, the recovery movement has attracted attention from both sides of the political spectrum. Recovery attracts both progressive activists and conservative politicians. The more liberally minded are drawn to its appreciation of diversity, and the more conservative minded are drawn to its libertarian strands and decreased costs. As an example of the latter, George Bush's President's New Freedom Commission put "recovery" at the heart of its recommendations for sweeping mental health reform (Hogan 2003, 1469; Sowers 2005).

The core features of the recovery movement involve a fundamental shift in psychiatry from a value structure of "experts know best" to one of "service-user control." As medical anthropologist and research scientist Kim Hopper summarizes, the recovery movement primarily concerns "reworking traditional power relationships, conferring distinctive expertise on service users, and rewriting the mandate of public mental health systems" (Hopper 2007, 868). To see how the recovery movement does this, consider the Substance Abuse and Mental Health Service Administration (SAMHSA) 2006 consensus conference on recovery. The conference brought together more than a hundred consumers, family members, clinicians, researchers, organizational representatives, and state and local public officials with the goal of defining and articulating the concepts of recovery. The SAMHSA statement they created begins with an overview that puts the move from experts-know-best to service-user control at its core: "Mental health recovery is a journey of healing and transformation enabling a person with a mental health problem to live a meaningful life in the community of his or her choice while striving to achieve his or her full potential" (SAMHSA 2006).

The statement goes on to outline ten fundamental components of recovery-oriented care: (1) self-direction, (2) individualized and person-centered, (3) empowerment, (4) holistic, (5) nonlinear, (6) strengths-based, (7) peer support, (8) respect, (9) responsibility, and (10) hope. These goals may seem at first glance like little more than good-quality care, but they are much more than that. As community psychiatrist and former senior medical adviser for SAMHSA Anita Everett put it: "Recovery is a critical paradigm shift for all individuals involved in the lives of persons with serious mental illnesses" (Everett 2005, 3).

To understand why recovery is such a paradigm shift in the direction of service-user control, we must note that the consensus participants did not see objective science as the primary lens through which to consider mental health. In recovery, the emphasis shifts from "objective knowledge" to "lived experience." Recovery approaches are less interested in the "truth" questions regarding mental illness and more interested in the experience of people who are different or who have troubles. Thus, the key questions from a recovery perspective move from "Where is it broken?" to "How can I be of help?"

In addition, once we move from a prime directive of "objective knowledge" to one of "lived experience," we simultaneously move away from reductionism toward holism and multiplicity. Mainstream scientific approaches tend in the direction of reductionism. Reduction can be valuable for some, as I've argued throughout this text, but for many in the recovery movement it has gone too far. By giving higher priority to lived experience, it is permissible, even desirable, to consider the big picture and to consider alternatives. Thus, under the principle of "holistic" care, the consensus statement emphasizes that "recovery encompasses an individual's whole life, including mind, body, spirit, and community." In addition, the tools of recovery may involve alternatives such as "complementary and naturalistic services" as well as deep attention to issues of "spirituality," "creativity," and "community involvement" that go far beyond the usual province of science (SAMHSA 2006).

The recovery movement makes a further paradigm shift toward lived experience, holism, and multiplicity by emphasizing the importance of social and political factors in mental health. The opening sentence of the consensus statement quoted above brings this message front and center: "Mental health recovery" means living "a meaningful life" in a community of choice. Recovery, therefore, is not simply about individuals. It involves finding and building mutual support communities and cultures that provide "a sense of belonging, supportive relationships, valued roles, and community" where people can "collectively and effectively speak for themselves about their needs, wants, desires, and aspirations" (SAMHSA 2006). Community psychiatrist Kenneth Thompson explains that these features of recovery speak to the critical importance of the principle of "empowerment." For Thompson, empowerment is so important to the recovery paradigm that the whole movement could arguably be called the "empowerment movement" (Thompson 2006).

This view is situated in a larger context than clinical care alone. From a recovery perspective this call to find and build community is about changing the social relations of difference. Recovery "not only benefits individuals with mental health disabilities . . . but also enriches the texture of American community life. America reaps the benefits of the contributions individuals with mental disabilities can make, ultimately becoming a stronger and healthier Nation" (SAMHSA 2006). If stigma excludes, this view insists on the mutual benefits and obligations of inclusion. As consumer, family member, and social worker Paulo del Vecchio succinctly puts it, because "stigma and discrimination are inexorably linked," the bottom line for recovery is "no justice, no recovery" (del Vecchio 2006, 646).

In all these dimensions, recovery creates a shift away from the centrality of "experts"—professionals, academics, researchers, codes of practice, training courses, and university departments. In the standard paradigm, "service users might be consulted and invited to comment on the models and the interventions and the research, but they are always recipients of expertise generated elsewhere" (Bracken 2007, 401). In contrast, in recovery approaches, service users are considered the true experts. They are the ones who most understand the challenges of psychic difference and psychic pain, sanism and exclusion, power and coercion, contexts and meanings, values and priorities, mental health care dysfunction and disinterest. This does not mean that recovery-oriented approaches reject professional services or contributions. It simply means that professional contributions become secondary rather than primary. As critical psychiatrist Patrick

Bracken put it: "The most radical implication of the recovery agenda, with its reversal of what is of primary and secondary significance, is the fact that when it comes to issues to do with values, meanings and relationships, it is users/survivors themselves who are the most knowledgeable and informed. When it comes to the recovery agenda, they are the real experts" (2007, 402).

Conclusion

Despite the recent support that consumer-oriented values have received from community psychiatry, it is too early to know how far the recovery movement will go in psychiatry. However far it goes, it is clear that the desire for consumer empowerment runs deep in the service-user community and many psychiatrists take this desire seriously. My point in describing this movement is to emphasize that just as bioethics opened the door to narrative medicine, both bioethics and the recovery movement open the door to narrative psychiatry. Both bioethics and the recovery movement call for clinicians who are comfortable with and who encourage empowered clients. They both call for clinicians who can empathically connect with clients' desires and preferences and who are willing to let the clients take the lead in making decisions. That, of course, does not mean that professionals have no role in recovery. Even with empowered consumers, there remains a place for professionals with skills needed to help people find their path to recovery.

What is important to see is that these professional skills, at their heart, are narrative skills. Narrative psychiatry creates clinicians who put the client's personal experience and preference at the forefront. And narrative psychiatry creates recovery-oriented clinicians who understand the many languages of psychic life. They are as comfortable talking about Yoga, creativity, and politics as they are neurotransmitters, cognitive distortions, and psychodynamics. Both the bioethics movement and the recovery movement make clear that many consumers wish for clinicians who have both of these skills.

CHAPTER TEN

Critical Reflections

THE EVIDENCE OF Mrs. Dutta's story and the efforts of bioethics and the recovery movement make a compelling case for adopting narrative approaches, but there are also many objections to putting narrative psychiatry into wider practice. It helps to work through these objections because responding to critics moves us beyond theory and creates space to consider more practical concerns. In addition, working through objections allows us to reweave our current ideas about psychiatry into a new narrative whole that can address many of the conceptual tension that arise in the practice of narrative psychiatry. In this section, I consider many of the common objections to narrative psychiatry.

Fiction Is Not Real

Some objectors to narrative psychiatry are concerned that narrative psychiatry relies *too much* on the evidence of fiction. Mrs. Dutta is not real, these objectors point out; she is fiction. Ivanov is not real either; he too is fiction. Fiction authors have no allegiance to "reality" when they create characters; they can do as they please. Authors imagine characters that can do all kinds of impossible things: characters who can fly, who can shoot spider webs out of their wrists, and who can travel back and forth in time. This tells us nothing about the real world and what real people can do. These objectors argue that there is no reason to take fiction seriously for understanding the real world. Chekhov and Divakaruni may write ambiguous stories, stories open to multiple interpretations, but so what. That does not mean that a real life Mrs. Dutta or a real-life Ivanov would be equally ambiguous. If Mrs. Dutta and Ivanov were real, there would be a real truth to their problems with real solutions.

Narrative psychiatrists respond that this objection harks back to the science wars we discussed in the last chapter. The objection rests on a sharp binary between "objective" and "subjective" and also between "fact" and "fiction." But there is a library of theoretical and philosophical work that troubles these binaries and shows how they create an array of problems. Sharp and rigid use of these binaries obscures the way that the "objective" world is always shaped by "subjective" frames (such as personal goals, cultural expectations, political interests, institutional practices, conceptual metaphors, and linguistic distinctions). And it misses the way that "fiction" contains real information that allows us to see and understand the world in new ways. People do not write or read fiction just for the possibilities of detached fantasy. They do it because fiction provides access to the author's imaginative view of reality. There is almost always some referential dimension to this imaginative view (Ricoeur 1977, 221). For psychiatry, a major part of the referential dimension is that fiction is an insight into the multiple dimensions of psychic life. This new information informs us that the problems people bring to the clinics are open to more than one explanation. To ignore this information just because it comes from literature makes no sense. It also leaves psychiatry out of touch with a basic wisdom needed for clinical work.

Where Are the Data?

A related objection argues that clinicians should not waste their time reading fiction and narrative theory; they should invest their resources in outcome studies and evidence-based research. "Sure," this objection goes, "there are lots of different approaches to psychiatric problems, but the only way to sort out which ones are effective is to do clinical trials." Narrative psychiatrists respond to this objection in two ways.

The first is simply to say yes, more empirical research is needed. As I've argued throughout, narrative psychiatrists have no reason to shy away from empirical research. Learning from fiction and interpretive philosophies does not preclude learning from empirical research. If empirical research makes a compelling argument in favor of a particular interpretation for a particular problem, narrative psychiatrists want to know about it. Narrative psychiatrists are as quick to refer people with pneumonia for antibiotic treatment as the next psychiatrist. And narrative psychiatrists make a point of helping their clients understand the data available for different options they might choose. For example, if Mrs. Dutta saw a narrative psychiatrist and the question of medications came up, the narrative psychiatrist would actually be much more explicit about the data on antidepressants than even more pure-minded biopsychiatrists (if we take Klein and Wender to be examples). Compared with Klein and Wender, narrative psychiatrists would spend time discussing the controversies in the literature. They would explain that some researchers are skeptical about the benefits of antidepressants and some are worried about potential risks involved.

In addition, narrative psychiatrists continue, they are hardly shy of data because many of the findings from empirical research support narrative perspectives. As discussed in Chapter 3, many studies comparing the efficacy of psychotherapies find that all therapeutic approaches do about the same. The Dodo bird verdict given to this finding ("everybody has won and all must have prizes") suggests that common factors may be more important than specific techniques in most therapeutic outcomes. Common factors include exposure to a kind and trusting therapeutic relationship, the comfort of the therapeutic rituals, the companionship and hope that flow from the therapeutic process, and the provision of a compelling and believable therapeutic rational. Narrative psychiatry, when done well, excels at all of these common factors because narrative psychiatrists puts the common factors of therapy in the foreground while remaining flexible and open to client preferences with regard to specific techniques.

That said, it is also true that the Dodo bird verdict remains controversial. Some argue that design flaws in the studies mask important differences between clients and therapies. As a result, some argue that the Dodo bird studies focus heavily on average outcomes rather than on particular conditions. Arkowitz and Lilienfeld explain this concern: "It is possible that although outcomes of various therapies may not differ, some clients may do better with one therapy, whereas other clients may do better with another" (Arkowitz and Lilienfeld 2006, 46). Narrative psychiatrists agree with this possibility. That is one of the main reasons for remaining flexible in their approach.

But even if research ends up supporting this possibility, as I discussed in Chapter 9, narrative psychiatry joins with values-based medicine to argue that science alone cannot fully decide for individuals which approach is "best" for them. Outcome studies may make useful claims in some situations and can sometimes provide assistance in thinking through options, but science is not the only factor. In addition, outcome studies face a major limitation in that the very idea of determining "which clients" go with "which therapy" depends on having pure diagnostic groups and pure therapeutic techniques. Most clients and most therapies are not so clean, and researchers who try to sharpen outcome studies often have to reject many of their recruited subjects.

Narrative psychiatry's second response to the call for empirical data as the best, and for some only, route to knowledge in psychiatry is to warn against idealizing science. Even though science has a role in psychiatric inquiry, narrative psychiatrists remind us that science does not come from nowhere and does not have extra human access to the world. Science is a human activity just like literature and interpretive theory. Science, like these other human activities, is therefore an open process. It is permeated by human interests, goals, and profiteering. Humans select the projects, the models, the methods, the meaning of the data, the definition of *peer* in peer review, and so on. All these human choices in science mean that findings from science cannot be mistaken for "objective truth" any more than can findings from literature or interpretive theory. Scientific findings may be useful and valuable, or they may be harmful and misleading. The latter is particularly true in times of excessive research funded by the pharmaceutical industry. As a result of the human side of science, science should be seen as a human tool, not something to idealize or devalue, and certainly not the only route to knowledge.

This Is "Philosophy Light"

Paradoxically, coming from the opposite direction, a call for greater rigor can also create objectors from literature and philosophy. These disciplinary humanities objectors argue that narrative psychiatry is theoretically and philosophically too thin. It rests on an insufficient awareness of fiction and too little interpretive philosophy. These objectors argue that if psychiatry is to take seriously the possibilities of fiction, it requires a much thicker engagement with the literature and philosophy. The difficulties of terms like *metaphor, plot, character,* and *point of view,* along with the difficulties of epistemology and ontology, have been only partially explored. And what about additional narrative elements like setting, dialogue, tone, and style? All these issues are highly relevant to the stories people tell about their troubles. Grounding narrative psychiatry in the work of Paul Ricoeur helps, but Ricoeur is only one philosopher, and even the richness of his work has only been hinted at in narrative psychiatry. In short, for these humanities scholars much more needs to be done in literature and philosophy to work through the conceptual issues in narrative psychiatry.

Narrative psychiatry's first response to these concerns is to agree. Yes, more work from the humanities is needed. Narrative psychiatry invites scholars in these domains to add their sophistication and insight to clinical work. That said, narrative psychiatry will never be a pure humanities discipline and must remain an interdisciplinary endeavor. Narrative psychiatry brings together insights from a variety of domains for the specific purpose of clinical work. Thus narrative psychiatry is an interdisciplinary scholarship that will always be too broad to completely satisfy disciplined critics from the humanities (or from the sciences). Disciplined critics must remember that disciplinary *depth of knowledge* is not necessarily superior to interdisciplinary *breadth of knowledge*. Both depth and breadth have their roles, and interdisciplinary work is as valuable as disciplinary work. The dangers of dilettantism in interdisciplinary work are real, but so are the dangers of overspecialization in disciplinary work.

Narrative Psychiatry Is Old Hat

The next objection to narrative psychiatry is the "nothing new" objection. Psychiatrists, this objection goes, are already good listeners and are already open to multiple dimensions of people's problems. Indeed, multiple dimensions to psychiatric problems is the whole point of George Engel's classic "biopsychosocial model." These objectors conclude that because most psychiatrists already listen carefully and because most adopt some version of the biopsychosocial model, narrative psychiatry adds little to what clinicians already do.

Narrative psychiatrists' first response to this objection is that they are not so sure about psychiatrists being "good listeners"—especially because more and more biopsychiatric research, education, and practice emphasize neuroscience, which tends to distance clinicians from the human part of their work. Psychiatrists trained in the times of psychoanalysis may have been good listeners, and yes, some of those traits remain in the profession. But there is little reason to believe this is still true or will remain true over time without ongoing support for the listening side of the work.

As for the biopsychosocial model, narrative psychiatrists respond by agreeing that it is more open than most other models. The biopsychosocial model does not simply consider biological variables or psychological variables or social variables; it considers at all three. Narrative psychiatrists remind us, however, that the "biopsychosocial model" is still a model and it too organizes clinical interpretations in a particular way. If we interpret Mrs. Dutta's sadness through the biopsychosocial model, we come up with a little biology, a little psychology, and a little family (and perhaps a little cross-cultural) tension. The story of Mrs. Dutta's sadness composed of a little biology, a little psychology, and a little family conflict is considerably different from one composed of genetics and neurotransmitters (as in a narrow biopsychiatry model). The first story is a broadly hybrid story, and the second is a purer narrative of biology. The biopsychosocial model is not the solution to interpretive diversity because both stories could be viable for Mrs. Dutta and the two stories cannot be collapsed.

Beyond this, the biopsychosocial model does little, if anything, with the creative, political, or spiritual aspects of human problems. Nor does it say anything about competing models within a single dimension—such as the alternatives between psychoanalysis and cognitive behavioral at the psychological level or the alternatives between family and political at the social level. It would be possible to modify the biopsychosocial model so that it included additional dimensions by expanding the model's definition of "psychology" and "social" (Lewis 2007). Similarly, one could even expand the biopsychosocial model to include narrative concerns. Both of these moves are possible because the phenomena of creativity, spirituality, and narration all take place somewhere within the psychological and social realm. But even if all these modifications were made, the result would be another "new" model—not the one true answer. An expanded biopsychosocial model would perhaps look very much like a narrative model. But even a narrative model is a model. One cannot assume it is superior to other models for all people at all times. It is an option, an invitation, not a necessity.

Narrative Psychiatry Is Too Broad

This discussion of the option, or invitation, of narrative psychiatry (rather than the necessity of it) is particularly relevant to critics who find narrative psychiatry too broad and prefer much more narrowly focused approaches. To take one example, critics from biopsychiatry argue that narrative psychiatry blurs the focus of their approach. These critics feel that biopsychiatry is superior to other approaches, and no amount of philosophy or reading of fiction will convince them otherwise.

For these critics, narrative psychiatrists can support single-minded perspectives if these perspectives can allow the caveat that their approach is best "for some therapists and for some clients." In other words, narrative psychiatrists can readily agree that medication approaches (or any other single-minded approach) may be best for certain person in a certain situation and that it is a completely viable option to choose one approach. That is in many ways the point of the exercise with Mrs. Dutta. Any one approach may work and could rationally be called "the best." Similarly, narrative psychiatrists support the value of any particular combination of options as well. Any two approaches (such as cognitive behavioral and medication) or any three approaches (such as psychoanalysis, Zen meditation, and political activism) might be the best for some clients in some situations. This is why narrative psychiatry comes close to eclectic psychiatry. A major difference is that narrative psychiatry adds considerable theoretical and philosophical sophistication to the usual versions of eclecticism.

You Can't Just Say Anything

Narrative psychiatry's openness to a variety of healing options is the kernel of another strong critique—the claim that narrative psychiatry is radically relativistic, that it is open to any and all interpretations, and that it provides no basis for making choices between different options. Here narrative psychiatrists respond by reminding these critics that narrative psychiatry does not claim an "anything goes" approach to interpretation. Different interpretations have different consequences, and therefore which interpretation, or which combination of interpretations, one chooses matters greatly. Also, because narrative psychiatrists follow Ricoeur and others who do not deny a referential dimension to narrative models, they are comfortable with the possibility that in some situations one model compared with another comes closer to describing the ultimate reality of the situation. Narrative psychiatry recommends moving beyond *either* "ultimate reality" *or* "worldview" metaphors for "world." When we move to a "world as a narrative perspective on ultimate reality" metaphor, there still remains a place for ultimate reality considerations.

The rub is that for narrative psychiatry questions of which consequences are best and which aspect of ultimate reality should be emphasized cannot be answered by the clinician. These questions must be answered by the client because, in the end, it is his or her life. Dialogue with clinicians can be immensely helpful for clients in making these decisions. But clients retain the autonomy to determine which understanding of their life gives them the most desired consequences. As for the question of which model best fits ultimate reality, narrative psychiatrists argue that this too must always remain a question of judgment, trial and error, and wisdom. Clinicians can help with these questions, but the decision is not theirs. Even conditions that may seem obvious to clinicians—such as autism or mental retardation—may turn out to be much more complicated for clients and their families. For these conditions a biological model may seem to be obvious to many. It may seem to "cut nature at its joints," and applying other models may seem "just plain wrong." Clinicians might feel confident that mental retardation cannot be cured with Zen meditation, and to a degree that may be true. But narrative psychiatrists argue that it is a mistake to get heavy handed about appeals to ultimate reality because it blocks the imagination. Other options may be surprising in the end. For example, if the goal is not "cure" of cognitive functioning but developing a sense of well-being, other models might be relevant. Zen meditation, for example, may come closer for some people than biology to the ultimate reality of mental retardation.

Narrative Psychiatry Is Just an Authority Trip

As this response highlights, narrative psychiatry works hard to avoid falling into a radical relativity critique and to show that it is not a sophomoric philosophy of "anything goes." This position leaves narrative psychiatry open to the opposite concern—that it is not relative enough and that it is too controlling. In other words, some critics argue that narrative psychiatry remains too narrow minded in the end. These critics point out that, for all its claim to openness and multiplicity, additional options are available for understanding human life that have hardly been mentioned. There are many models from different cultures and subcultures that have not been discussed. There is also the possibility that individuals may come up with completely novel solutions to life situations not captured in any of the models available. And finally, all this talk of narrative identity makes it seem that people who have no such story to organize their lives are somehow inferior or inadequate.

Narrative psychiatrists appreciate these critiques and the opportunity to make clear that, yes, there are many models and approaches that have not been addressed. Any number of additional possibilities are available and potentially useful. Also, narrative psychiatrists agree that people can create their own approach independent of any existing approaches. The link between metaphor and model means that it is as possible to develop a new model as it is to develop a new metaphor. Following Ricoeur, a new metaphor, sometimes called a live metaphor, contrasts with a dead metaphor in that a dead metaphor has become naturalized through extended use. "Depression is a chemical imbalance" was once a live metaphor and might still be for someone who has not heard it. But for most people it has become so naturalized that it seems like a literal statement. The same is true to some degree for most of the approaches we discussed. But people are not confined to dead metaphors. In the process of narrating their lives, they may create new ones. As Ricoeur puts it, language creates infinite possibilities out of finite resources (Ricoeur 1991c, 65).

As for the critique that narrative psychiatry overvalues the well-storied self, this seems to a problem of emphasis more than a fundamental difficulty. Contemporary fiction is full of stories, so-called postmodern narratives, in which the characters and the plots are fragmented and disjointed without any obvious narrative coherence. On the surface, it might seem that these postmodern stories are "against narrativity." Indeed, philosopher Galen Strawson wrote a compelling essay that reaches a similar perspective to argue against what he calls the *descriptive narrative thesis* and the *normative narrative thesis* (Strawson 2004). The *descriptive thesis* is the empirical claim that people use narrative to organize their experience. Strawson finds this thesis showing up in authors like Jerome Brunner who claim that the "self is a perpetually rewritten story." The *normativity thesis* argues that, whether people do or do not live their lives as story, the good life requires a good story. A richly narrative outlook, in other words, is "essential to a well-lived life, to true and full personhood" (2004, 423).

Strawson argues against both theses. For him, there are deeply "non-narrative" people who experience life episodically—one thing after another—rather than through a well-narrated plot. In addition, there are good ways to live life non-narratively, and the good life does not require a good story. To think otherwise, Strawson agues, is to "close down important avenues of thought, impoverish our grasp of ethical possibilities, [and] needlessly and wrongly distress those who do not fit their model" (2004, 429).

For narrative psychiatrists, Strawson's arguments provide an important check against taking narrative too seriously, but they do not necessitate an "against narrativity" polemic. If "narrativity" is defined broadly rather than narrowly, it becomes expansive enough to include "non-narrative" or episodic lives. Narrative psychiatrists certainly agree with Strawson that there should not be a heavy-handed insistence that the narratives people tell about themselves be coherent or that their narrative identities should be whole. But this does not require a polemic against narrative because episodic and fragmented narratives are after all still narratives.

Narrative Psychiatry Is Not Practical

Another, often strongly voiced, objection to narrative psychiatry is that it is just not practical. These objectors point out that there are many cases in which psychiatrists do not, and should not, rely on the client to make decisions. What if clients are a danger to themselves or others? What if they are incompetent? What if they need to be committed to a hospital against their will or even medicated over objection? Narrative psychiatrists respond that these complicated legal and ethical issues do not prohibit narrative approaches to understanding clinical problems. It is true, of course, that narrative psychiatrists, like other psychiatrists, must work within the local standards of care. Sometimes these standards require narrative psychiatrists to interrupt the narrative process to make quick, and relatively unilateral, judgments and interventions. However, that says little about how clients may ultimately understand their situation or the meaning of these interruptions. Clients may have to go to the hospital against their will because the narrative psychiatrist interpreted them as "mentally ill" and a "danger to self or others," but that interpretation is hardly final. Ongoing narrative work may amend it tremendously. The client may eventually conclude that it was the psychiatrist who was a danger to others by forcing him or her in the hospital, and as more information emerges, the psychiatrist might even agree.

Practicality critics go further. Even if narrative psychiatry can negotiate emergency issues, they argue, it remains unpractical on a day-to-day level. There is just not time, these critics argue, for clinicians to work through all of a person's narrative options. Clients want solutions and they want them fast. They cannot afford to wait, and they do not have insurance that will pay for them to dawdle with fanciful ideas about narrative. Narrative psychiatrists respond that for most clients it works the other way around. The most efficient clinical care is care that tunes into clients' preferences. If the clinician tries to anticipate these preferences without narrative tools, she or he will often slow the process by going down needless blind alleys.

Furthermore, narrative psychiatrists respond to these practical "resource" critiques by pointing out that time and money are not just physical constraints, they are also elements of a story. If clients decide that they do not want to consider their options, that is still a narrative. For example, a client might say, "I was feeling rotten and went to see a psychiatrist. She let me know that there are many approaches to my problems and she would be happy to spend a few sessions discussing these options or she could simply recommend something. I was feeling so bad, plus my money was so tight, I decided to do whatever she recommended." In other words, even if clients decide not to explore their options, it matters that they have been told about them. There is nothing unpractical about this. It is, or should be, the minimum of informed choice. It also allows clients to decide later that, should they desire, they can change their mind and consider their options more fully.

In addition, narrative psychiatrists respond to the practicality critique that narrative choices permeate the clinical encounter so much that it is impossible to avoid them. These options do not stop once a client and psychiatrist have started down a particular path. No matter which approach they take, there will be a myriad of additional narrative choices along the way. And, once again, the most efficient way to deal with the many forks in the road will be through narrative tools. This is true even if a psychiatrist and client embark on the most medical of psychiatric treatments: a trial of medications. Even here, a host of narrative options remain regarding which medications to take, whether to add more, whether to live with the side effects, and so on. All of these are more than strictly "medical decisions." They are deeply ethical decisions about what kind of person the client wants to be and what kind of life he or she wants to live.

Narrative Psychiatry Treats Biopsychiatry as Reductive

Biopsychiatry, as I have discussed, has been the subject of much critique because of its reductionism tendencies. Throughout this book, I have argued that despite its reduction, biopsychiatry still is a valuable paradigm for understanding aspects of human psychic life. As I have pointed out, all ways of knowing are ultimately reductive, so reduction in and of itself is not a critique of biopsychiatry.

But some object that this take on biopsychiatry misses the point with regard to biological models. They point out that recent work in neuroscience has moved beyond reductive approaches and has become highly expansive. Expansive neuroscience has developed to the point that there is now a neuroscience of such wide-ranging human activities as positive emotion, meaning making, interpersonal relations, empathy, creativity, psychoanalysis, politics, ethics, meditation, and even theology. There is no reason to believe this expansive trend in neuroscience won't continue to develop such that there will be a scientific interpretation of the neuroanatomical functions and plastic changes in everything human, including narrative. If this is true, why do we need to respect all these many approaches? Why do we even need narrative? If neuroscience can expand to consider all things human, wouldn't neuroscience be all we need?

Narrative psychiatry agrees that the expansive trend in neuroscience will likely grow and that expansive neurosciences will create new hybrid languages—which mix brain talk with many other kinds of talk. However, these new hybrid brain languages, like other languages, must be understood as not "better" but "different." Neuroethics, neuropolitics, neurotheology, or neuropsychoanalysis are not inherently better than ethics politics, theology, or psychoanalysis. Combining previously nonbrain languages with brain languages creates new insights but also covers over other insights, which means that some of the richness of the previous perspective is lost. Many will be attracted to the new insights and the supposed new legitimacy that comes from brain talk and brain research. Narrative psychiatrists have no trouble appreciating the appeals of brain talk combined with other kinds of languages. When these new ways of talking, thinking, and being are valuable and preferred for particular people and particular goals, narrative psychiatrists will happily support the use of this emergent language.

But not everyone will gravitate to these new languages. For some, all this brain talk will not be compelling. They will feel like more is lost than gained, and they will see this emergent language as manipulative. They will see the new brain talk as today's "biobabble," which is taking the place of yesterday's "psychobabble" (Cameron 2007). For them, other ways of thinking about human life outside neuroscience will be more appealing. Narrative approaches allow psychiatrists to use emergent neurolanguages when they are helpful but also to avoid idealizing them or insisting on them.

I Don't Like Narrative Psychiatry

The final objection I will address is one to which narrative psychiatry has no response. Some people object to narrative psychiatry because they just do not like it. Some psychiatrists and some clients do not like literature, the humanities, cultural studies, or any of this "mushy" stuff. They prefer only nonfiction and hard science. Others enjoy literature and do not mind thinking about meaning and theory, but they see it as a hobby or recreation—nothing to do with clinical concerns. None of these people respond well to narrative psychiatry. They prefer having nothing to do with it, and they wish to keep going as before: they like the metaphor for "world" as ultimate reality, they prefer single truths over multiple truths, and they wish to keep it that way.

This objection has no response because narrative psychiatry can only respect the objection as a preferred worldview. A non-narrative approach to psychiatry is a legitimate way to organize the world with many good consequences. Narrative psychiatry could argue against this worldview by saying that people who do not like narrative are still telling stories and using narrative devices whether they accept it or not. But narrative psychiatry has no grounds to play trumps with other points of view. Of course, narrative psychiatry can make this metanarrative argument in favor of narrative. Indeed, I used a similar argument in some of my comments above. But I'm not dogmatic about it. Indeed, a "nothing but stories" metanarrative is not all that different from a biopsychiatrist saying that narrative is "nothing but neurochemistry." I do not have to be persuaded by that claim just because it is a metanarrative claim. Within a narrative frame, metanarrative arguments remain arguments, not ultimate appeals to the universal truth. If objectors are not persuaded, there are few grounds from a narrative perspective to insist on a claim to deeper knowledge.

However, even though narrative psychiatry does not appeal to the trump of "truth," it does not unilaterally disarm itself. Yes, narrative psychiatry gives up trumps, but it also takes away the trump position from the non-narrative position. Single-minded and often scientistic approaches may still be legitimate in psychiatry, but they can no longer have absolute authority. Single-minded approaches must recognize that there are many other ways, and they must play fair with others. They cannot rule out narrative psychiatry by imperial decree; they must join the fray of communal decision making. They must accept, in other words, that the question of how to balance scientistic approaches with other approaches is a human question and ultimately a political question, not a science question alone.

Conclusion

Despite the many objections to narrative psychiatry, the time for a narrative turn has arrived in psychiatry. Narrative is deeply consistent with recent trends in bioethics and recovery to increase consumers' involvement in their care. In addition, narrative approaches already have a solid place psychiatry's two sister disciplines—medicine and psychotherapy. Finally, narrative thinking is a cornerstone of most intellectual thought. The field of psychiatry cannot and should not ignore these historical trends. Even if some psychiatrists reject a narrative turn, a significant part of the field must join the fold of history.

The timing of this narrative turn makes sense not only because of events surrounding psychiatry but also because of events within psychiatry. This past century saw psychiatry swing from biopsychiatry to psychoanalysis and then back again. But as we move further into a new century, it makes little sense for psychiatry to keep this pendulum going. It is time to move beyond dichotomous thinking, and it is time to let go of endless swings between a brainless psychiatry and a meaningless psychiatry.

Now is the ideal time to make this move because now is the moment when biopsychiatry has reached such a dominant position that psychoanalysis is about to fade away completely. Not only that, biopsychiatry itself has started to generate considerable critique. These two phenomena are connected because the remnants of psychoanalysis protected biopsychiatry from its more crassly scientistic side. During the early years of biopsychiatry, psychoanalysis provided a bank of meaning-based wisdom that continued to influence the field. Psychoanalysis could do this because, even though it often talked in terms of science, it worked much more like one of the humanities. Psychoanalysis based its thinking on an interpretive practice and drew extensive insights from literature and the arts. But as psychoanalysis has faded in favor of biopsychiatry, this repository of meaning-centered psychiatry has faded with it.

This loss exposes the limits of biopsychiatry. By itself, biopsychiatry has few tools for understanding the interpretive aspects of clinical encounters. Substituting cognitive behavioral approaches for psychoanalysis is not a sufficient solution because cognitive behavioral approaches, like biospsychiatry, rest primarily on the logics of science. Cognitive behavioral approaches do not take sufficient interest in the humanities and the arts to keep psychiatry true to its human side. Returning to psychoanalysis is also not the solution because psychoanalysis itself never truly developed its interpretive tools. Psychoanalysis never took seriously enough its human side to join systematically with the humanities. This was Karl Jaspers's critique of psychoanalysis early in the past century, and it continues to be relevant for psychoanalysis.

The solution for psychiatry is to bring back the key insights of Jaspers. He was right about psychoanalysis, and he was right about psychiatry more broadly. Psychiatry has always been, and always will be, a practice that is about both causes and meanings (and the many philosophical complications of this conceptual divide). By embracing Jaspers's wisdom, narrative psychiatry agrees with scholars in philosophy and psychiatry who follow in Jaspers's footsteps to call for a "renaissance in philosophy of psychiatry" (Fulford, Morris, Sadler, and Stanghellini 2003b, 1). Narrative psychiatry simply extends this renaissance beyond philosophy to include the humanities, cultural studies, and the arts. The decline of psychoanalysis, although a loss for psychiatry, is also an opportunity to further develop the meaning side of psychiatry because it brings psychiatry back to the moment of Jaspers's intervention.

By taking advantage of this moment, narrative psychiatry is poised to help psychiatry join more systematically with the "other side" of campus, the side often designated as the "arts and humanities." Jaspers understood that it never made sense to develop psychiatry without this side of campus. The dabbling that clinical psychoanalysis did in the humanities, while helpful, was never sufficient. Clinical psychoanalysis resided primarily in institutions and was therefore was also largely cut off from ongoing work in literature, philosophy, and cultural study. Now is the ideal moment for psychiatry to both self-correct from the limits of biopsychiatry *and* go further than clinical psychoanalysis could do in developing the arts and humanities side of psychiatry. Now is the moment to bring the different sides of psychiatry together with the different sides of campus. Narrative psychiatry opens the door to this kind of deeply nuanced practice of psychiatry. The next step is for significant numbers in the field to go through that door.

"Mrs. Dutta Writes a Letter"

By Chitra Divakaruni

When the alarm goes off at 5:00 a.m., buzzing like a trapped wasp, Mrs. Dutta has been lying awake for quite a while. She still has difficulty sleeping on the Perma Rest mattress that Sagar and Shyamoli, her son and daughter-in-law, have bought specially for her, though she has had it now for two months. It is too American-soft, unlike the reassuring solid copra ticking she used at home. *But this is home now,* she reminds herself. She reaches hurriedly to turn off the alarm, but in the dark her fingers get confused among the knobs, and the electric clock falls with a thud to the floor. Its angry metallic call vibrates through the walls of her room, and she is sure it will wake everyone. She yanks frantically at the wire until she feels it give, and in the abrupt silence that follows she hears herself breathing, a sound harsh and uneven and full of guilt.

Mrs. Dutta knows, of course, that this ruckus is her own fault. She should just not set the alarm. She does not need to get up early here in California, in her son's house. But the habit, taught her by her mother-in-law when she was a bride of seventeen, *A good wife wakes before the rest of the household,* is one she finds impossible to break. How hard it was then to pull her unwilling body away from the sleep-warm clasp of her husband, Sagar's father, whom she had just learned to love; to stumble to the kitchen that smelled of stale garam masala and light the coal stove so that she could make morning tea for them all—her parents-in-law, her husband, his two younger brothers, and the widowed aunt who lived with them.

After dinner, when the family sits in front of the TV, she tries to tell her grandchildren about those days. "I was never good at starting that stove—the smoke stung my eyes, making me cough and cough. Breakfast was never ready on time, and my mother-in-law—oh, how she scolded me, until I was in tears. Every night I'd pray to Goddess Durga, please let me sleep late, just one morning!"

"Mmmm," Pradeep says, bent over a model plane.

"Oooh, how awful," Mrinalini says, wrinkling her nose politely before she turns back to a show filled with jokes that Mrs. Dutta does not understand.

"That's why you should sleep in now, Mother," Shyamoli says, smiling at her from the recliner where she sits looking through the *Wall Street Journal*. With her legs crossed so elegantly under the shimmery blue skirt she has changed into after work, and her unusually fair skin, she could pass for an American, thinks Mrs. Dutta, whose own skin is as brown as roasted cumin. The thought fills her with an uneasy pride.

From the floor where he leans against Shyamoli's knee, Sagar adds, "We want you to be comfortable, Ma. To rest. That's why we brought you to America."

In spite of his thinning hair and the gold-rimmed glasses that he has recently taken to wearing, Sagar's face seems to Mrs. Dutta still that of the boy she used to send off to primary school with his metal tiffin box. She remembers how he crawled into her bed on stormy monsoon nights, how when he was ill, no one else could make him drink his barley water. Her heart lightens in sudden gladness because she is really here, with him and his children in America. "Oh, Sagar," she says, smiling, "now you're talking like this! But did you give me a moment's rest while you were growing up?" And she launches into a description of childhood pranks that has him shaking his head indulgently while disembodied TV laughter echoes through the room.

But later he comes into her bedroom and says, a little shamefaced, "Mother, please don't get up so early in the morning. All that noise in the bathroom—it wakes us up, and Molli has such a long day at work . . ."

And she, turning a little so that he won't see her foolish eyes filling with tears, as though she were a teenage bride again and not a woman well over sixty, nods her head, *yes, yes.*

Waiting for the sounds of the stirring household to release her from the embrace of her Perma Rest mattress, Mrs. Dutta repeats the 108 holy names of God. *Om Keshavaya Namah, Om Narayanaya Namah, Om Madhavaya Namah.* But underneath she is thinking of the bleached-blue aerogram from Mrs. Basu that has been waiting unanswered on her bedside table all week, filled with news from home. Someone robbed the Sandhya jewelry store. The bandits had guns, but luckily no one was hurt. Mr. Joshi's daughter, that sweet-faced child, has run away with her singing teacher. Who would've thought it? Mrs. Barucha's daughter-in-law had one more baby girl. Yes, their fourth. You'd think they'd know better than to keep trying for a boy. Last Tuesday was Bangla Bandh, another labor strike, everything closed down, not even the buses running. But you can't really blame them, can you? After all, factory workers have to eat too. Mrs. Basu's tenants, whom she'd been trying to evict forever, finally moved out. Good riddance, but you should see the state of the flat.

At the very bottom Mrs. Basu wrote, *Are you happy in America?*

Mrs. Dutta knows that Mrs. Basu, who has been her closest friend since they both moved to Ghoshpara Lane as young brides, cannot be fobbed off with descriptions of Fisherman's Wharf and the Golden Gate Bridge, or even with anecdotes involving grandchildren. And so she has been putting off her reply, while in her heart family loyalty battles with insidious feelings of—but she turns from them quickly and will not name them even to herself.

Now Sagar is knocking on the children's doors—a curious custom, this, children being allowed to close their doors against their parents. With relief Mrs. Dutta gathers up her bathroom things. She has plenty of time. Their mother will have to rap again before Pradeep and Mrinalini open their doors and stumble out. Still, Mrs. Dutta is not one to waste the precious morning. She splashes cold water on her face and neck (she does not believe in pampering herself), scrapes the night's gumminess from her tongue with her metal tongue cleaner, and brushes vigorously, though the minty toothpaste does not leave her mouth feeling as clean as does the bittersweet neem stick she's been using all her life. She combs the knots out of her hair. Even at her age it is thicker and silkier than her daughter-in-law's permed curls. *Such vanity,* she scolds her reflection, *and you a grandmother and a widow besides.* Still, as she deftly fashions her hair into a neat coil, she remembers how her husband would always compare it to monsoon clouds.

She hears a sudden commotion outside.

"Pat! Minnie! What d'you mean you still haven't washed up? I'm late to work every morning nowadays because of you kids."

"But Mom, *she's* in there. She's been there forever . . ." Mrinalini says.

Pause. Then, "So go to the downstairs bathroom."

"But all our stuff is here," Pradeep says, and Mrinalini adds, "It's not fair. Why can't *she* go downstairs?"

A longer pause. Mrs. Dutta hopes that Shyamoli will not be too harsh with the girl. But a child who refers to elders in that disrespectful way ought to be punished. How many times did she slap Sagar for something far less, though he was her only one, the jewel of her eye, come to her after she had been married for seven years and everyone had given up hope? Whenever she lifted her hand to him, her heart was pierced through and through. Such is a mother's duty.

But Shyamoli only says, in a tired voice, "That's enough! Go put on your clothes, hurry!"

The grumblings recede. Footsteps clatter down the stairs. Inside the bathroom Mrs. Dutta bends over the sink, fists tight in the folds of her sari. Hard with the pounding in her head to think what she feels most—anger at the children for their rudeness, or at Shyamoli for letting them go unrebuked. Or is it shame she feels (but why?), this burning, acid and indigestible, that coats her throat in molten metal?

It is 9:00 a.m., and the house, after the flurry of departures, of frantic "I can't find my socks" and "Mom, he took my lunch money" and "I swear I'll leave you kids behind if you're not in the car in exactly one minute," has settled into its quiet daytime rhythms.

Busy in the kitchen, Mrs. Dutta has recovered her spirits. Holding on to grudges is too exhausting, and besides, the kitchen—sunlight spilling across its countertops while the refrigerator hums reassuringly in the background—is her favorite place.

Mrs. Dutta hums too as she fries potatoes for alu dum. Her voice is rusty and slightly off-key. In India she would never have ventured to sing, but with everyone gone the house is too quiet, all that silence pressing down on her like the heel of a giant hand, and the TV voices, with their strange foreign accents, are no help at all. As the potatoes turn golden-brown, she permits herself a moment of nostalgia for her Calcutta kitchen—the new gas stove she bought with the birthday money Sagar sent, the scoured-shiny brass pots stacked by the meat safe, the window with the lotus-pattern grille through which she could look down on white-uniformed children playing cricket after school. The mouthwatering smell of ginger and chili paste, ground fresh by Reba, the maid, and, in the evening, strong black Assam tea brewing in the kettle when Mrs. Basu came by to visit. In her mind she writes to Mrs. Basu: *Oh, Roma, I miss it all so much. Sometimes I feel that someone has reached in and torn out a handful of my chest.*

But only fools indulge in nostalgia, so Mrs. Dutta shakes her head clear of images and straightens up the kitchen. She pours the half-drunk glasses of milk down the sink, though Shyamoli has told her to save them in the refrigerator. But surely Shyamoli, a girl from a good Hindu family, doesn't expect her to put contaminated *jutha* things with the rest of the food. She washes the breakfast dishes by hand instead of letting them wait inside the dishwasher till night, breeding germs. With practiced fingers she throws an assortment of spices into the blender: coriander, cumin, cloves, black pepper, a few red chiles for vigor. No stale bottled curry powder for her. *At least the family's eating well since I arrived,* she writes in her mind. *Proper Indian food, puffed-up chapatis, fish curry in mustard sauce, and real pulao with raisins and cashews and ghee—the way you taught me, Roma—instead of Rice-a-roni.* She would like to add, *They love it,* but thinking of Shyamoli, she hesitates.

At first Shyamoli was happy enough to have someone take over the cooking. "It's wonderful to come home to a hot dinner," she'd say. Or "Mother, what crispy papads, and your fish curry is out of this world." But recently she has taken to picking at her food, and once or twice from the kitchen Mrs. Dutta has caught wisps of words, intensely whispered: "cholesterol," "all putting on weight," "she's spoiling you." And though Shyamoli always says no when the children ask if they can have burritos from the freezer instead, Mrs. Dutta suspects that she would really like to say yes.

The children. A heaviness pulls at Mrs. Dutta's entire body when she thinks of them. Like so much in this country, they have turned out to be—yes, she might as well admit it—a disappointment.

For this she blames, in part, the Olan Mills portrait. Perhaps it was foolish of her to set so much store by a photograph, especially one taken years ago. But it was such a charming scene—Mrinalini in a ruffled white dress with her arm around her brother, Pradeep chubby and dimpled in a suit and bow tie, a glorious autumn forest blazing red and yellow behind them. (Later Mrs. Dutta was saddened to learn that the forest was merely a backdrop in a studio in California, where real trees did not turn such colors.)

The picture had arrived, silver-framed and wrapped in a plastic sheet filled with bubbles, with a note from Shyamoli explaining that it was a Mother's Day gift. (A strange concept, a day set aside to honor mothers. Did the sahibs not honor their mothers the rest of the year, then?) For a week Mrs. Dutta could not decide where it should be hung. If she put it in the drawing room, visitors would be able to admire her grandchildren, but if she put it on the bedroom wall, she would be able to see the photo last thing before she fell asleep. She finally opted for the bedroom, and later, when she was too ill with pneumonia to leave her bed for a month, she was glad of it.

Mrs. Dutta was accustomed to living on her own. She had done it for three years after Sagar's father died, politely but stubbornly declining the offers of various relatives, well-meaning and otherwise, to come and stay with her. In this she surprised herself as well as others, who thought of her as a shy, sheltered woman, one who would surely fall apart without her husband to handle things for her. But she managed quite well. She missed Sagar's father, of course, especially in the evenings, when it had been his habit to read to her the more amusing parts of the newspaper while she rolled out chapatis. But once the grief receded, she found she enjoyed being mistress of her own life, as she confided to Mrs. Basu. She liked being able, for the first time ever, to lie in bed all evening and read a new novel of Shankar's straight through if she wanted, or to send out for hot eggplant pakoras on a rainy day without feeling guilty that she wasn't serving up a balanced meal.

When the pneumonia hit, everything changed.

Mrs. Dutta had been ill before, but those illnesses had been different. Even in bed she'd been at the center of the household, with Reba coming to find out what should be cooked, Sagar's father bringing her shirts with missing buttons, her mother-in-law, now old and tamed, complaining that the cook didn't brew her tea strong enough, and Sagar running in crying because he'd had a fight with the neighbor boy. But now she had no one to ask her querulously, *Just how long do you plan to remain sick?* No one waited in impatient exasperation for her to take on her duties again. No one's life was inconvenienced the least bit by her illness.

Therefore she had no reason to get well.

When this thought occurred to Mrs. Dutta, she was so frightened that her body grew numb. The walls of the room spun into blackness; the bed on which she lay, a vast four-poster she had shared with Sagar's father since their wedding, rocked like a dinghy caught in a storm; and a great hollow roaring reverberated inside her head. For a moment, unable to move or see, she thought, *I'm dead.* Then her vision, desperate and blurry, caught on the portrait. *My grandchildren.* With some difficulty she focused on the bright, oblivious sheen of their faces, the eyes so like Sagar's that for a moment heartsickness twisted inside her like a living thing. She drew a shudder of breath into her aching lungs, and the roaring seemed to recede. When the afternoon post brought another letter from Sagar—*Mother, you really should come and live with us. We worry about you all alone in India, especially when you're sick like this*—she wrote back the same day, with fingers that still shook a little, *You're right: my place is with you, with my grandchildren.*

But now that she is here on the other side of the world, she is wrenched by doubt. She knows the grandchildren love her—how can it be otherwise among family? And she loves them, she reminds herself, even though they have put away, somewhere in the back of a closet, the vellum-bound *Ramayana for Young Readers* that she carried all the way from India in her hand luggage. Even though their bodies twitch with impatience when she tries to tell them stories of her girlhood. Even though they offer the most transparent excuses when she asks them to sit with her while she chants the evening prayers. *They're flesh of my flesh, blood of my blood,* she reminds herself. But sometimes when she listens, from the other room, to them speaking on the phone, their American voices rising in excitement as they discuss a glittering, alien world of Power Rangers, Metallica, and Spirit Week at school, she almost cannot believe what she hears.

Stepping into the back yard with a bucket of newly washed clothes, Mrs. Dutta views the sky with some anxiety. The butter-gold sunlight is gone, black-bellied clouds have taken over the horizon, and the air feels still and heavy on her face, as before a Bengal storm. What if her clothes don't dry by the time the others return home?

Washing clothes has been a problem for Mrs. Dutta ever since she arrived in California.

"We can't, Mother," Shyamoli said with a sigh when Mrs. Dutta asked Sagar to put up a clothesline for her in the back yard. (Shyamoli sighed often nowadays.

Perhaps it was an American habit? Mrs. Dutta did not remember that the Indian Shyamoli, the docile bride she'd mothered for a month before putting her on a Pan Am flight to join her husband, pursed her lips in quite this way to let out a breath at once patient and exasperated.) "It's just not *done*, not in a nice neighborhood like this one. And being the only Indian family on the street, we have to be extra careful. People here sometimes—" She broke off with a shake of her head. "Why don't you just keep your dirty clothes in the hamper I've put in your room, and I'll wash them on Sunday along with everyone else's."

Afraid of causing another sigh, Mrs. Dutta agreed reluctantly. She knew she should not store unclean clothes in the same room where she kept the pictures of her gods. That would bring bad luck. And the odor. Lying in bed at night she could smell it distinctly, even though Shyamoli claimed that the hamper was airtight. The sour, starchy old-woman smell embarrassed her.

She was more embarrassed when, on Sunday afternoons, Shyamoli brought the laundry into the family room to fold. Mrs. Dutta would bend intently over her knitting, face tingling with shame, as her daughter-in-law nonchalantly shook out the wisps of lace, magenta and sea-green and black, that were her panties, placing them next to a stack of Sagar's briefs. And when, right in front of everyone, Shyamoli pulled out Mrs. Dutta's crumpled, baggy bras from the heap, she wished the ground would open up and swallow her, like the Sita of mythology.

Then one day Shyamoli set the clothes basket down in front of Sagar.

"Can you do them today, Sagar?" (Mrs. Dutta, who had never, through the forty-two years of her marriage, addressed Sagar's father by name, tried not to wince.) "I've *got* to get that sales report into the computer by tonight."

Before Sagar could respond, Mrs. Dutta was out of her chair, knitting needles dropping to the floor.

"No, no, no, clothes and all is no work for the man of the house. I'll do it." The thought of her son's hands searching through the basket and lifting up his wife's— and her own—underclothes filled her with horror.

"Mother!" Shyamoli said. "This is why Indian men are so useless around the house. Here in America we don't believe in men's work and women's work. Don't I work outside all day, just like Sagar? How'll I manage if he doesn't help me at home?"

"I'll help you instead," Mrs. Dutta ventured.

"You don't understand, do you, Mother?" Shyamoli said with a shaky smile. Then she went into the study.

Mrs. Dutta sat down in her chair and tried to understand. But after a while she gave up and whispered to Sagar that she wanted him to teach her how to run the washer and dryer.

"Why, Mother? Molli's quite happy to—"

"I've got to learn it . . ." Her voice was low and desperate as she rummaged through the tangled heap for her clothes.

Her son began to object and then shrugged. "Oh, very well. If it makes you happy."

But later, when she faced the machines alone, their cryptic symbols and rows of gleaming knobs terrified her. What if she pressed the wrong button and flooded the entire floor with soapsuds? What if she couldn't turn the machines off and they kept going, whirring maniacally, until they exploded? (This had happened on a TV show just the other day. Everyone else had laughed at the woman who jumped up and down, screaming hysterically, but Mrs. Dutta sat stiff-spined, gripping the armrests of her chair.) So she has taken to washing her clothes in the bathtub when she is alone. She never did such a chore before, but she remembers how the village washerwomen of her childhood would beat their saris clean against river rocks. And a curious satisfaction fills her as her clothes hit the porcelain with the same solid wet *thunk*.

My small victory, my secret.

This is why everything must be dried and put safely away before Shyamoli returns. Ignorance, as Mrs. Dutta knows well from years of managing a household, is a great promoter of harmony. So she keeps an eye on the menacing advance of the clouds as she hangs up her blouses and underwear, as she drapes her sari along the redwood fence that separates her son's property from the neighbor's, first wiping the fence clean with a dish towel she has secretly taken from the bottom drawer in the kitchen. But she isn't worried. Hasn't she managed every time, even after that freak hailstorm last month, when she had to use the iron from the laundry closet to press everything dry? The memory pleases her. In her mind she writes to Mrs. Basu: *I'm fitting in so well here, you'd never guess I came only two months back. I've found new ways of doing things, of solving problems creatively. You would be most proud if you saw me.*

When Mrs. Dutta decided to give up her home of forty-five years, her relatives showed far less surprise than she had expected. "Oh, we all knew you'd end up in America sooner or later," they said. She had been foolish to stay on alone so long after Sagar's father, may he find eternal peace, passed away. Good thing that boy of hers had come to his senses and called her to join him. Everyone knows a wife's place is with her husband, and a widow's is with her son.

Mrs. Dutta had nodded in meek agreement, ashamed to let anyone know that the night before she had awakened weeping.

"Well, now that you're going, what'll happen to all your things?" they asked.

Mrs. Dutta, still troubled over those traitorous tears, had offered up her household effects in propitiation. "Here, Didi, you take this cutwork bedspread.

Mashima, for a long time I have meant for you to have these Corning Ware dishes; I know how much you admire them. And Boudi, this tape recorder that Sagar sent a year back is for you. Yes, yes, I'm quite sure. I can always tell Sagar to buy me another one when I get there."

Mrs. Basu, coming in just as a cousin made off triumphantly with a bone-china tea set, had protested. "Prameela, have you gone crazy? That tea set used to belong to your mother-in-law."

"But what'll I do with it in America? Shyamoli has her own set—"

A look that Mrs. Dutta couldn't read flitted across Mrs. Basu's face. "But do you want to drink from it for the rest of your life?"

"What do you mean?"

Mrs. Basu hesitated. Then she said, "What if you don't like it there?"

"How can I not like it, Roma?" Mrs. Dutta's voice was strident, even to her own ears. With an effort she controlled it and continued. "I'll miss my friends, I know—and you most of all. And the things we do together—evening tea, our walk around Rabindra Sarobar Lake, Thursday night Bhagavad Gita class. But Sagar—they're my only family. And blood is blood, after all."

"I wonder," Mrs. Basu said drily, and Mrs. Dutta recalled that though both of Mrs. Basu's children lived just a day's journey away, they came to see her only on occasions when common decency dictated their presence. Perhaps they were tight-fisted in money matters too. Perhaps that was why Mrs. Basu had started renting out her downstairs a few years earlier, even though, as anyone in Calcutta knew, tenants were more trouble than they were worth. Such filial neglect must be hard to take, though Mrs. Basu, loyal to her children as indeed a mother should be, never complained. In a way, Mrs. Dutta had been better off, with Sagar too far away for her to put his love to the test.

"At least don't give up the house," Mrs. Basu was saying. "You won't be able to find another place in case . . ."

"In case what?" Mrs. Dutta asked, her words like stone chips. She was surprised to find that she was angrier with Mrs. Basu than she'd ever been. Or was she afraid? *My son isn't like yours,* she'd been on the verge of spitting out. She took a deep breath and made herself smile, made herself remember that she might never see her friend again.

"Ah, Roma," she said, putting her arm around Mrs. Basu. "You think I'm such an old witch that my Sagar and my Shyamoli will be unable to live with me?"

Mrs. Dutta hums a popular Tagore song as she pulls her sari from the fence. It's been a good day, as good as it can be in a country where you might stare out the window for hours and not see one living soul. No vegetable vendors with enormous wicker baskets balanced on their heads, no knife sharpeners with their distinctive call—*scissors-knives-choppers, scissors-knives-choppers*—to bring the children running. No peasant women with colorful tattoos on their arms to sell you cookware in exchange for your old silk saris. Why, even the animals that frequented Ghoshpara Lane had personality—stray dogs that knew to line up outside the kitchen door just when the leftovers were likely to be thrown out; the goat that maneuvered its head through the garden grille, hoping to get at her dahlias; cows that planted themselves majestically in the center of the road, ignoring honking drivers. And right across the street was Mrs. Basu's two-story house, which Mrs. Dutta knew as well as her own. How many times had she walked up the stairs to that airy room, painted sea-green and filled with plants, where her friend would be waiting for her?

What took you so long today, Prameela? Your tea is cold already.

Wait till you hear what happened, Roma. Then you won't scold me for being late—

Stop it, you silly woman, Mrs. Dutta tells herself severely. *Every single one of your relatives would give an arm and a leg to be in your place, you know that. After lunch you're going to write a nice letter to Roma telling her exactly how delighted you are to be here.*

From where Mrs. Dutta stands, gathering up petticoats and blouses, she can look into the next yard. Not that there's much to see—just tidy grass and a few pale blue flowers whose name she doesn't know. Two wooden chairs sit under a tree, but Mrs. Dutta has never seen anyone using them. *What's the point of having such a big yard if you're not even going to sit in it?* she thinks. Calcutta pushes itself into her mind again, with its narrow, blackened flats where families of six and eight and ten squeeze themselves into two tiny rooms, and her heart fills with a sense of loss she knows to be illogical.

When she first arrived in Sagar's home, Mrs. Dutta wanted to go over and meet her next-door neighbors, maybe take them some of her special sweet rasogollahs, as she'd often done with Mrs. Basu. But Shyamoli said she shouldn't. Such things were not the custom in California, she explained earnestly. You didn't just drop in on people without calling ahead. Here everyone was busy; they didn't sit around chatting, drinking endless cups of sugar-tea. Why, they might even say something unpleasant to her.

"For what?" Mrs. Dutta had asked disbelievingly, and Shyamoli had said, "Because Americans don't like neighbors to"—here she used an English phrase—"invade their privacy." Mrs. Dutta, who didn't fully understand the word *privacy,* because there was no such term in Bengali, had gazed at her daughter-in-law in some bewilderment. But she understood enough not to ask again. In the following months, though, she often looked over the fence, hoping to make contact. People were people, whether in India or in America, and everyone appreciated a friendly face. When Shyamoli was as old as Mrs. Dutta, she would know that too.

Today, just as she is about to turn away, out of the corner of her eye Mrs. Dutta notices a movement. At one of the windows a woman is standing, her hair a sleek gold like that of the TV heroines whose exploits baffle Mrs. Dutta when she tunes in to an afternoon serial. She is smoking a cigarette, and a curl of gray rises lazily, elegantly, from her fingers. Mrs. Dutta is so happy to see another human being in the middle of her solitary day that she forgets how much she disapproves of smoking, especially in women. She lifts her hand in the gesture she has seen her grandchildren use to wave an eager hello.

The woman stares back at Mrs. Dutta. Her lips are a perfect painted red, and when she raises her cigarette to her mouth, its tip glows like an animal's eye. She does not wave back or smile. Perhaps she is not well? Mrs. Dutta feels sorry for her, alone in her illness in a silent house with only cigarettes for solace, and she wishes the etiquette of America did not prevent her from walking over with a word of cheer and a bowl of her fresh-cooked alu dum.

Mrs. Dutta rarely gets a chance to be alone with her son. In the morning he is in too much of a hurry even to drink the fragrant cardamom tea that she (remembering how as a child he would always beg for a sip from her cup) offers to make him. He doesn't return until dinnertime, and afterward he must help the children with their homework, read the paper, hear the details of Shyamoli's day, watch his favorite TV crime show in order to unwind, and take out the garbage. In between, for he is a solicitous son, he converses with Mrs. Dutta. In response to his questions she assures him that her arthritis is much better now; no, no, she's not growing bored being at home all the time; she has everything she needs—Shyamoli has been so kind. But perhaps he could pick up a few aerograms on his way back tomorrow? She obediently recites for him an edited list of her day's activities, and smiles when he praises her cooking. But when he says, "Oh, well, time to turn in, another working day tomorrow," she feels a vague pain, like hunger, in the region of her heart.

So it is with the delighted air of a child who has been offered an unexpected gift that she leaves her half-written letter to greet Sagar at the door today, a good hour before Shyamoli is due back. The children are busy in the family room doing homework and watching cartoons (mostly the latter, Mrs. Dutta suspects). But for once she doesn't mind, because they race in to give their father hurried hugs and then race back again. And she has him, her son, all to herself in a kitchen filled with the familiar, pungent odors of tamarind sauce and chopped coriander leaves.

"Khoka," she says, calling him by a childhood name she hasn't used in years, "I could fry you two-three hot-hot luchis, if you like." As she waits for his reply, she can feel, in the hollow of her throat, the rapid thud of her heart. And when he says yes, that would be very nice, she shuts her eyes tight and takes a deep breath, and it is as though merciful time has given her back her youth, that sweet, aching urgency of being needed again.

Mrs. Dutta is telling Sagar a story.

"When you were a child, how scared you were of injections! One time, when the government doctor came to give us compulsory typhoid shots, you locked yourself in the bathroom and refused to come out. Do you remember what your father finally did? He went into the garden and caught a lizard and threw it in the bathroom window, because you were even more scared of lizards than of shots. And in exactly one second you ran out screaming—right into the waiting doctor's arms."

Sagar laughs so hard that he almost upsets his tea (made with real sugar, because Mrs. Dutta knows it is better for her son than that chemical powder Shyamoli likes to use). There are tears in his eyes, and Mrs. Dutta, who had not dared to hope that he would find her story so amusing, feels gratified. When he takes off his glasses to wipe them, his face is oddly young, not like a father's at all, or even a husband's, and she has to suppress an impulse to put out her hand and rub away the indentations that the glasses have left on his nose.

"I'd totally forgotten," Sagar says. "How can you keep track of those old, old things?"

Because it is the lot of mothers to remember what no one else cares to, Mrs. Dutta thinks. *To tell those stories over and over, until they are lodged, perforce, in family lore. We are the keepers of the heart's dusty corners.*

But as she starts to say this, the front door creaks open, and she hears the faint click of Shyamoli's high heels. Mrs. Dutta rises, collecting the dirty dishes.

"Call me fifteen minutes before you're ready to eat, so that I can fry fresh luchis for everyone," she tells Sagar.

"You don't have to leave, Mother," he says.

Mrs. Dutta smiles her pleasure but doesn't stop. She knows that Shyamoli likes to be alone with her husband at this time, and today, in her happiness, she does not grudge her this.

"You think I've nothing to do, only sit and gossip with you?" she mock-scolds. "I want you to know I have a very important letter to finish."

Somewhere behind her she hears a thud—a briefcase falling over. This surprises her. Shyamoli is always careful with it, because it was a gift from Sagar when she was finally made a manager in her company.

"Hi!" Sagar calls, and when there's no answer, "Hey, Molli, you okay?"

Shyamoli comes into the room slowly, her hair disheveled as though she has been running her fingers through it. Hot color blotches her cheeks.

"What's the matter, Molli?" Sagar walks over to give her a kiss. "Bad day at work?" Mrs. Dutta, embarrassed as always by this display of marital affection, turns toward the window, but not before she sees Shyamoli move her face away.

"Leave me alone." Her voice is low, shaking. "Just leave me alone."

"But what is it?" Sagar says with concern.

"I don't want to talk about it right now." Shyamoli lowers herself into a kitchen chair and puts her face in her hands. Sagar stands in the middle of the room, looking helpless. He raises his hand and lets it fall, as though he wants to comfort his wife but is afraid of what she might do.

A protective anger for her son surges inside Mrs. Dutta, but she moves away silently. In her mind-letter she writes, *Women need to be strong, not react to every little thing like this. You and I, Roma, we had far worse to cry about, but we shed our tears invisibly. We were good wives and daughters-in-law, good mothers. Dutiful, uncomplaining. Never putting ourselves first.*

A sudden memory comes to her, one she hasn't thought of in years—a day when she scorched a special kheer dessert. Her mother-in-law had shouted at her, "Didn't your mother teach you anything, you useless girl?" As punishment she refused to let Mrs. Dutta go with Mrs. Basu to the cinema, even though *Sahib, Bibi aur Ghulam*, which all Calcutta was crazy about, was playing, and their tickets were bought already. Mrs. Dutta had wept the entire afternoon, but before Sagar's father came home, she washed her face carefully with cold water and applied *kajal* to her eyes so that he wouldn't know.

But everything is getting mixed up, and her own young, trying-not-to-cry face blurs into another—why, it's Shyamoli's—and a thought hits her so sharply in the chest that she has to hold on to her bedroom wall to keep from falling. *And what good did it do? The more we bent, the more people pushed us, until one day we'd forgotten that we could stand up straight. Maybe Shyamoli's the one with the right idea after all . . .*

Mrs. Dutta lowers herself heavily onto her bed, trying to erase such an insidious idea from her mind. Oh, this new country, where all the rules are upside down, it's confusing her. The space inside her skull feels stirred up, like a pond in which too many water buffaloes have been wading. Maybe things will settle down if she can focus on the letter to Roma.

Then she remembers that she has left the half-written aerogram on the kitchen table. She knows she should wait until after dinner, after her son and his wife have sorted things out. But a restlessness—or is it defiance?—has taken hold of her. She is sorry that Shyamoli is upset, but why should she have to waste her evening because of that? She'll go get her letter—it's no crime, is it? She'll march right in and pick it up, and even if Shyamoli stops in mid-sentence with another one of those sighs, she'll refuse to feel apologetic. Besides, by now they're probably in the family room, watching TV.

Really, Roma, she writes in her head, as she feels her way along the unlighted corridor, *the amount of TV they watch here is quite scandalous. The children too, sitting for hours in front of that box like they've been turned into painted dolls, and then talking back when I tell them to turn it off.* Of course she will never put such blasphemy into a real letter. Still, it makes her feel better to be able to say it, if only to herself.

In the family room the TV is on, but for once no one is paying it any attention. Shyamoli and Sagar sit on the sofa, conversing. From where she stands in the corridor, Mrs. Dutta cannot see them, but their shadows—enormous against the wall where the table lamp has cast them—seem to flicker and leap at her.

She is about to slip unseen into the kitchen when Shyamoli's rising voice arrests her. In its raw, shaking unhappiness it is so unlike her daughter-in-law's assured tones that Mrs. Dutta is no more able to move away from it than if she had heard the call of the *nishi,* the lost souls of the dead, the subject of so many of the tales on which she grew up.

"It's easy for you to say 'Calm down.' I'd like to see how calm *you'd* be if she came up to you and said, 'Kindly tell the old lady not to hang her clothes over the fence into my yard.' She said it twice, like I didn't understand English, like I was a savage. All these years I've been so careful not to give these Americans a chance to say something like this, and now—"

"Shhh, Shyamoli, I *said* I'd talk to Mother about it."

"You always say that, but you never *do* anything. You're too busy being the perfect son, tiptoeing around her feelings. But how about mine? Aren't I a person too?"

"Hush, Molli, the children . . ."

"Let them hear. I don't care anymore. Besides, they're not stupid. They already know what a hard time I've been having with her. You're the only one who refuses to see it."

In the passage Mrs. Dutta shrinks against the wall. She wants to move away, to hear nothing else, but her feet are formed of cement, impossible to lift, and Shyamoli's words pour into her ears like fire.

"I've explained over and over, and she still does what I've asked her not to—throwing away perfectly good food, leaving dishes to drip all over the counter-tops. Ordering my children to stop doing things I've given them permission to do. She's taken over the entire kitchen, cooking whatever she likes. You come in the door and the smell of grease is everywhere, in all our clothes even. I feel like this isn't my house anymore."

"Be patient, Molli. She's an old woman, after all."

"I know. That's why I tried so hard. I know having her here is important to you. But I can't do it any longer. I just can't. Some days I feel like taking the kids and leaving." Shyamoli's voice disappears into a sob.

A shadow stumbles across the wall to her, and then another. Behind the weatherman's nasal tones, announcing a week of sunny days, Mrs. Dutta can hear a high, frightened weeping. The children, she thinks. This must be the first time they've seen their mother cry.

"Don't talk like that, sweetheart." Sagar leans forward, his voice, too, anguished. All the shadows on the wall shiver and merge into a single dark silhouette.

Mrs. Dutta stares at that silhouette, the solidarity of it. Sagar and Shyamoli's murmurs are lost beneath the noise in her head, a dry humming—like thirsty birds, she thinks wonderingly. After a while she discovers that she has reached her room. In darkness she lowers herself onto her bed very gently, as though her body were made of the thinnest glass. Or perhaps ice—she is so cold. She sits for a long time with her eyes closed, while inside her head thoughts whirl faster and faster until they disappear in a gray dust storm.

When Pradeep finally comes to call her for dinner, Mrs. Dutta follows him to the kitchen, where she fries luchis for everyone, the perfect circles of dough puffing up crisp and golden as always. Sagar and Shyamoli have reached a truce of some kind: she gives him a small smile, and he puts out a casual hand to massage the back of her neck. Mrs. Dutta shows no embarrassment at this. She eats her dinner. She answers questions put to her. She laughs when someone makes a joke. If her face is stiff, as though she had been given a shot of Novocain, no one notices. When the table is cleared, she excuses herself, saying she has to finish her letter.

Now Mrs. Dutta sits on her bed, reading over what she wrote in the innocent afternoon.

Dear Roma,

Although I miss you, I know you will be pleased to hear how happy I am in America. There is much here that needs getting used to, but we are no strangers to adjusting, we old women. After all, haven't we been doing it all our lives?

Today I'm cooking one of Sagar's favorite dishes, alu dum. It gives me such pleasure to see my family gathered around the table, eating my food. The children are still a little shy of me, but I am hopeful that we'll soon be friends. And Shyamoli, so confident and successful—you should see her when she's all dressed for work. I can't believe she's the same timid bride I sent off to America just a few years ago. But Sagar, most of all, is the joy of my old age. . . .

With the edge of her sari Mrs. Dutta carefully wipes a tear that has fallen on the aerogram. She blows on the damp spot until it is completely dry, so the pen will not leave a telltale smudge. Even though Roma would not tell a soul, she cannot risk it. She can already hear them, the avid relatives in India who've been waiting for something just like this to happen. *That Dutta-ginni, so set in her ways, we knew she'd never get along with her daughter-in-law.* Or, worse, *Did you hear about poor Prameela? How her family treated her? Yes, even her son, can you imagine?*

This much surely she owes to Sagar.

And what does she owe herself, Mrs. Dutta, falling through black night with all the certainties she trusted in collapsed upon themselves like imploded stars, and only an image inside her eyelids for company? A silhouette—man, wife, children, joined on a wall—showing her how alone she is in this land of young people. And how unnecessary.

She is not sure how long she sits under the glare of the overhead light, how long her hands clench themselves in her lap. When she opens them, nail marks line the soft flesh of her palms, red hieroglyphs—her body's language, telling her what to do.

Dear Roma, Mrs. Dutta writes,

I cannot answer your question about whether I am happy, for I am no longer sure I know what happiness is. All I know is that it isn't what I thought it to be. It isn't about being needed. It isn't about being with family either. It has something to do with love, I still think that, but in a different way than I believed earlier, a way I don't have the words to explain. Perhaps we can figure it out together, two old women drinking cha in your downstairs flat (for I do hope you will rent it to me on my return) while around us gossip falls—but lightly, like summer rain, for that is all we will allow it to be. If I'm lucky—and perhaps, in spite of all that has happened, I am—the happiness will be in the figuring out.

Pausing to read over what she has written, Mrs. Dutta is surprised to discover this: now that she no longer cares whether tears blotch her letter, she feels no need to weep.

NOTES

Preface

1. Throughout this book I use the terms *psychiatry* and *psychiatrists*; however, much of this material will be relevant for mental health workers more broadly. I welcome readers from outside psychiatry to consider these ideas.

2. Cultural studies of psychiatry may be seen as part of a larger genre, which Davis and Morris call "biocultures." See Davis and Morris 2007 for an articulation of the larger genre. For a review of this material, see Lewis 2009.

Chapter One: Listening to Chekhov

1. Many argue that the chemical imbalance model is a distortion of contemporary biopsychiatry (Lacasse and Leo 2005). But even if we accept this argument, it does not change the underlying disease logics at the core of biological psychiatry. See Helen Mayberg's discussion of limbic-cortical disregulation for an updated and sophisticated version of the neuropathology of depression (Mayberg 2004).

2. These numbers were calculated using drug sales data from IMS Health by Graham Aldred for the Alliance for Human Research Protection (AHRP) (www .arhp.org). AHRP is a well-known citizens' watchdog organization that brings public attention to human rights issues associated with biotech research and usage. For the details of Aldred's analysis, see Aldred 2004.

3. Breggin 1991; Caplan 1995; Farber 1993; Valenstein 1998.

4. Useful resources for understanding Chekhov's life and background include Chekhov 1997, 2004; Coope 1997; Finke 2005; Hingley 1976; and Rayfield 1997.

5. Because of the uniqueness of Chekhov's multiple positions, William Carlos Williams (also a master of literature and medicine) was correct when he told a young medical student looking for advice in understanding the subtleties of medicine to "read Chekhov, read story after story of his" (Coles 2002, xii). Contemporary physician Robert Norman says much the same thing when he tells fellow doctors, "I recommend you dive in [to Chekhov's writings] with abandon, soak

up the visions of Chekhov, and you will emerge the better person" (Norman 2005).

6. For a review of these portrayals from a medical perspective, see Coope 1997, chap. 2.

7. Although Kramer does not mention examples, it is certainly true that others in the medical humanities community interpret Ivanov in a similar way. Both Coope and Callahan also see Ivanov as clinically or biologically depressed. See Coope 1997, 34–38, and Coulehan 1997.

8. For an extended version of this argument, see Kramer 2005. Here, Kramer follows suit with his *Ivanov* review, using strategic polemic to claim that depression must be seen as a medical disease. He catalogs an array of contemporary scientific research that shows how depression disrupts brain functioning, damages the heart, and alters personal perspective. Kramer minimizes any complications of this interpretation to make the extreme claim that contemporary medical research demands that there be no alternative perspective on depression beyond a disease model.

9. See also Friedland 1964, 130.

10. For an excellent discussion of Bakhtin's concepts of "voice" and "polyphony" as applied to Chekhov and medicine, see Puustinen 1999, 2000. See also Kathy Popkin's discussion of Chekhov's frequent strategy of staging an incident and then providing two separate perspectives on it, "one that regards the incident as utterly trivial, barely worth mentioning, while the other discerns the maximal degree of catastrophe in the same event" (Popkin 1993, 38).

11. Subsequent references are cited parenthetically in the text with act, scene, and line numbers.

12. There is some evidence that Chekhov himself was not disposed to an environmental interpretation. Indeed, Chekhov explains in a letter that one of his early motivations for the play was to demolish all talk of Russia's superfluous men—the very Ivanov types that were so common in Russian literature at the time and who were generally understood to be suffering from a kind of social paralysis (see Chekhov 2004, 175). Gilman argues, however, that Chekhov's motivations may have changed in the course of writing the play. Although he at first wished to dispose of environmental explanations for Russia's "superfluous men," during the process of writing the play "he steadily transformed it into something much richer and far less thematically local" (Gilman 1995, 40). This interpretation would account for Chekhov's inclusion of general anomie in *Ivanov*'s setting, and it would account for including Sasha's outburst that diagnoses all the men in the area.

13. For a discussion of "dogmatism" in contemporary psychiatry, see Ghaemi 2003. Ghaemi concludes, based on an analysis of psychiatric practice, that ap-

proximately "64% of psychiatrists are dogmatists" (301). It is important to add that the cocksure self-confidence of psychiatry is bigger than individual psychiatrists. Even if many individual psychiatrists are plenty humble about their models, there remains an impression of certainty emanating from the field that comes from the sea of marketing and advertising devoted to promoting biomedical models. One is unlikely see a pharmaceutical advertisement that says "here is one way to understand and approach your troubles" (unless, of course, that line was to be rhetorically more persuasive in some contexts). The effect of this relentless hype about medical models easily creates the impression that the field is foolishly overconfident in its interpretations—just as Dr. Lvov turns out to be in Chekhov's play.

14. For a discussion of *DSM*-led heavy-handedness in psychiatric interpretations, see Wood 2004.

15. For an excellent collection of Chekhov's portrayals of clinicians, see Coulehan 2002.

16. See Greenhalgh 1999 for an attempt to reconcile the ambiguities of narrative medicine with the dictates of positivist medicine.

17. See Freud 1958. Freud uses the phrase "working through" to articulate the slow and often painful process of applying insight and meaning to the minutia of daily life. To use a more contemporary theorist of subjectivity, this "working through" may also be seen as a kind of Foucauldian "technology of the self" (Foucault 1988b, 16). The "working through" of the story is similar to what Michel Foucault means when he says that practices of the self are a kind of askesis, a form of training. It requires work and dedication to inhabit them. Askesis, Foucault summarizes, is "an exercise of self upon the self by which one tries to work out one's self and to attain a certain mode of being" (Foucault 1988a, 2). This approach to subjectivity links well to other theoretical work in the humanities such as Pierre Bourdieu's use of "habitus," Deleuze and Guatarri's "becoming," and Judith Butler's "performativity." For further references and discussions of these theorists of subjectivity, see Du Gay, Evans, and Redman 2000; Hall and Du Gay 1996; and Mansfield 2000.

18. Using language from postmodern theory, we can add that narrative multiplicity sidesteps the usual modernist dichotomy of realism verses relativism. It allows psychiatrists to embrace a flexible postpsychiatric ontology of *semiotic realism* and an epistemology of *pluridimensional consequences*.

By an ontology of semiotic realism, I mean to suggest that there is a real world out there that grounds our ideas and that our ideas are in touch with. However, the specific points of contact are determined by the semiotic relations from which our ideas are structured. These semiotic relations are relative to given narrative communities and traditions of thought. Semiotic realism rejects rigid ontologies of realism and relativism because it contains insights from both. Semiotic realism understands that knowledge articulations are grounded in the real world, but how and why they are grounded remain relative to a diverse multiplicity of narrative communities.

The related postpsychiatric epistemology of pluridimensional consequences combines the French poststructural insights with those of the American pragmatists. Roland Barthes uses the phrase "pluri-dimensional order" to articulate the way that specific languages always remain too limited to capture the world in total (Barthes 1982, 465). Despite this limitation, all linguistic communities do evoke, engage, and negotiate the world through some element of grounding or contact. Languages do not fully mirror or correspond to the world in all the world's complexity, but languages do make real connections with the world. For the American pragmatists, different connections with the world yield different *consequences* for practice and for lived experience. From this perspective, the best knowledge is that which leads to the best consequences in practice.

For an extended discussion of these postmodern terms, see Lewis 2006b, 18–37.

19. For an additional discussion of pluralism and psychiatry, see Ghaemi 2003. Ghaemi's and my analyses are similar in that they both rely on the work of American pragmatic philosophy. They differ in that my work combines pragmatism with insights from literary theory and poststructuralism.

Chapter Two: Narrative Medicine

1. Rutherford and Hellerstein provide a fascinating example of this relative trend in psychiatry compared with medicine. They analyzed the presence of humanities-style articles in psychiatry and internal medicine journals from 1950 to 2000. They found that in psychiatry journals humanities-related articles decreased from a peak of 17% in 1970 to a low of 2% in 2000. During the same period, humanities articles in internal medicine journals roughly doubled, from 5% to 11%. In short, humanities publications dramatically decreased over time in psychiatry journals while they more than doubled in internal medicine journals (Rutherford and Hellerstein 2008).

Chapter Three: Narrative Approaches to Psychotherapy

1. See Arkowitz and Lilienfeld 2006 for a good overview of debates surrounding psychotherapy research.

2. See Hubble, Duncan, and Miller 1999 for an extensive discussion of the implications of the Dodo bird verdict for psychotherapy.

3. See www.postmodernpsychology.com.

4. See Flax 1990.

5. This point will become clearer when I discuss values-based medicine in Chapter 9.

6. As I mentioned earlier, one way to sidestep the rigid binary between realism and relativism is through postmodern terms of semiotic realism and pluridimensional consequences (Lewis 2006b, 20–21). Narrative theory's focus on metaphor brings out related insights.

7. For an extended discussion of this concept, see Bachelor and Harvath 1999.

Chapter Four: Narrative Psychiatry

1. This story I'm telling—of sharp swings in U.S. psychiatry from biopsychiatry to psychoanalysis and back again—is told using broad strokes. Although it fits well with the mainstream of psychiatry, there have been and continue to be intermediary positions that integrate the models or hold the models in tension. Beyond the work of Jaspers (and often inspired by his legacy), some examples include Robert Coles's literary approaches, George Engel's "biopsychosocial model," Nassir Ghaemi's "pluralistic psychiatry," Paul McHugh and Phillip Slavney's "perspectives of psychiatry," and Adolph Meyer's "psychobiology" (Coles 1975; Engel 1977; Ghaemi 2003; McHugh and Slavney 1998; Meyer 1957). I leave out these intermediary positions in my broad overview because they have never had a major foothold in the field. Impressively, the perspectives approach of McHugh and Slavney has had considerable longevity at the Johns Hopkins University—and in that way is far ahead of its time (McHugh 1992). And, nationally, Engel's biopsychosocial model came the closest to gaining wide acceptance. But I agree with Ghaemi that even though many psychiatrists follow the biopsychosocial model in theory, they lean heavily toward biopsychiatry or psychoanalysis in practice (Ghaemi 2003, 21).

It would have been possible to have told this story of psychiatry differently and to foreground these additional options in psychiatry. Indeed, each of these intermediary alternatives has elements of what I am calling "narrative psychiatry." None of them does exactly what I mean by "narrative psychiatry," but I could have told this story by highlighting these alternatives as early moves toward narrative. But that would have made for a much longer story.

2. See Chapter 9 for further discussion of the recovery movement.

3. Interestingly, Coles's relation to psychiatry mirrors my own in some ways, except that it starts a little earlier. Coles trained in psychiatry when psychoanalysis was as dominant—and, for some, as dogmatic—as biopsychiatry has become today. Coles turned away from psychoanalysis toward more literary and storied approaches because of this dogma. Coles would later have the same reaction to

biopsychiatry that he once had to psychoanalysis. For Coles, when either psycho-analysis or biopsychiatry becomes too dominant, they drown out the many other elements of human stories.

4. Mainstream medicine leaves the disease/illness distinction intact by focusing almost exclusively on disease—to the point that the personal experience of illness all too often becomes lost in the clinical encounter. Narrative medicine, as we have seen, intervenes in medicine at exactly this point. Narrative medicine, similar to earlier reforms in medicine such as the biopsychosocial model and person-centered medicine, reminds mainstream medicine that it deals with more than pathophysiology; it deals with a whole persons. But though narrative medicine includes the patient's experience much more effectively than mainstream medicine, usually even narrative medicine does not have to trouble the disease/illness distinction. For the most part, narrative medicine can work with an additive logic with regard to this distinction. For narrative medicine, disease is important *and also* so is illness. In this formula, even in narrative medicine the distinction between disease and illness stays intact. This remains true when narrative physicians prescribe psychiatric medications because the point of narrative medicine is not to give psychiatric medications. The point is to tune into the unique personal experience of patients.

Narrative psychotherapy integration also does not usually need to trouble the distinction between disease and illness. For the most part, narrative psychotherapy integration focuses on experience and illness. Integrative psychotherapists, like most psychotherapists, would generally agree with Freud that people's biological constitution matters, but they would also agree with his decision to bracket biology and keep the focus of psychotherapy on psychological, or experiential, variables. Thus, in psychotherapy, the experience of suffering, the person's illness, becomes the primary focus of attention. Narrative psychotherapy integration follows suit with psychotherapy in this area by also staying focused on illness. Narrative psychotherapy integration adds that narrative tools and concepts may be helpful in understanding a person's illness and the identifications he or she makes during recovery. But, in general, even narrative psychotherapy integration, like psychotherapy more broadly, remains focused on illness, which allows it to leave disease/illness distinction undisturbed.

Chapter Five: Mrs. Dutta and the Literary Case

1. This does not mean that the thin stories clinicians tell are "bad" for all purposes. Indeed, I argued in Chapter 1 the value of reductive, or thin, stories for helping people understand their lives. They are just "bad" as a source of narrative psychiatry case studies.

Chapter Six: Mainstream Stories I

1. Other good sources for comparing clinical models include Corsini and Wedding 2005 and Gurman and Messer 2003.

2. Subsequent references are cited parenthetically in the text by page.

3. Although the authors take a non-narrative approach, a good overview of contemporary psychoanalytic models of depression can be found in Busch, Rudden, and Shapiro 2004. In contrast to a narrative approach, these psychoanalysts attempt to distill a single psychoanalytic model for depression out of the many psychoanalytic models that have been proposed. I would argue instead that any of the psychoanalytic models (including the one that Busch, Rudden, and Shapiro come up with) could continue to be helpful in the right circumstances.

Chapter Seven: Mainstream Stories II

1. Subsequent references are cited parenthetically in the text by page.

Chapter Eight: Alternative Stories

1. Subsequent references are cited parenthetically in the text by page.

Chapter Nine: Doing Narrative Psychiatry

1. This discussion assumes Mrs. Dutta is not a candidate for hospitalization. See the next chapter for a consideration of emergency situations, the issue of danger to self, and the question of involuntary hospitalization.

2. In discussing a related point, Tallman and Bohart argue for restorying the "hero" in psychotherapeutic encounters (Tallman and Bohart 1999). Typical narratives of psychotherapy place the therapists as the "hero"—the one who initiates change and saves the day. But, based on a reading of psychotherapy research, Tallman and Bohart argue for a complete reversal of the hero roles. The client is the hero. The therapist is at best a sidekick.

REFERENCES

Adams, P. 2000. Childism as vestiges of infanticide. *Journal of American Academy of Psychoanalysis* 28:541–56.

Alcoff, L. 2005. Foucault's philosophy of science: Structures of truth/structures of power. In G. Gutting, ed., 211–223. *Continental philosophy of science*. London: Blackwell.

Aldred, G. 2004. An analysis of the use of Prozac, Paxil, and Zoloft in USA, 1988–2002. Alliance for Research Protection. www.ahrp.org/risks/usSSRIuse0604.pdf (accessed January 2, 2006).

American Psychiatric Association. 1980. *Diagnostic and statistical manual of mental disorders,* 3d ed. Washington, DC: American Psychiatric Association Press.

———. 1995. *Diagnostic and statistical manual of mental disorders,* 4th ed. Washington, DC: American Psychiatric Association Press.

Andreasen, N. 1984. *The broken brain: The biological revolution in psychiatry.* New York: Harper and Row.

Andreasen, N., and Black, D. 1995. *Introductory textbook of psychiatry.* Washington, DC: American Psychiatric Press.

Angell, M. 2005. *The truth about drug companies: How they deceive us and what to do about it.* New York: Random House.

Angus, L., and McLeod. J. 2004. Toward an integrative framework for understanding the role of narrative in psychotherapy process. In L. Angus and J. McLeod, eds., *Handbook of narrative and psychotherapy: Practice, theory and research,* 367–374. Thousand Oaks, CA: Sage Publications.

Antonuccio, D., Burns, D., and Danton, W. 2002. Antidepressants: A triumph of marketing over science? *Prevention and Treatment* 5. www.journals.apa.org/prevention/volume5/toc-jul15-02.html (accessed June 2, 2005).

Arkowitz, H., and Lilienfeld, S. 2006. Psychotherapy on trial. *Scientific American Mind,* April/May: 42–49.

Bachelor, A., and Horvath, A. 1999. The therapeutic relationship. In M. Hubble, B. Duncan, and S. Miller, eds., *The heart and soul of change: What works in therapy,* 133–178. Washington, DC: American Psychological Association.

Bakhtin, M. 1994. *The Bakhtin reader: Selected writings of Bakhtin, Medvedev, Voloshinov*. Edited by P. Morris. London: Edward Arnold.

Barker, P. 1986. *Basic family therapy*, 2d ed. New York: Oxford University Press.

Barthes, R. 1982. Inaugural lecture, College de France. In S. Sontag, ed., *A Barthes reader*, 457–78. New York: Hill and Wang.

Beck, A., and Newman, C. 2005. Cognitive therapy. In B. Sadock and V. Sadock, eds., *Kaplan and Sadock's comprehensive textbook of psychiatry*, 8th ed., 2596–2611. Philadelphia: Lippincott Williams and Wilkins.

Beck, A., Rush, J., Shaw, B., and Emery, G. 1979. *Cognitive therapy of depression*. New York: Guilford Press.

Beck, A., and Weishaar, M. 2005. Cognitive therapy. In R. Corsini and D. Wedding, eds., *Current Psychotherapies*, 7th ed., 238–69. Belmont, CA: Brooks/Cole–Thomson.

Becvar, D., and Becvar, R. 2003. *Family therapy: A systemic integration*, 5th ed. Boston: Allyn and Bacon.

Bell, M. S. 1997. *Narrative design: Working with imagination, craft, and form*. New York: W. W. Norton.

Bordo, S. 1993. *Unbearable weight: Feminism, Western culture, and the body*. Berkeley: University of California Press.

Bracken, P. 2007. Beyond models, beyond paradigms: The radical interpretation of recovery. In P. Stasney and P. Lehmann, eds., *Alternatives beyond psychiatry*, 400–402. Berlin: Peter Lehman Publishing.

Bracken, P., and Thomas, P. 2005. *Postpsychiatry: Mental health in postmodern world*. Oxford: Oxford University Press.

Breggin, P. 1991. *Toxic psychiatry: Why therapy, empathy, and love must replace the drugs, electroshock, and biochemical theories of the "New Psychiatry."* New York: St. Martin's Press.

Brendel, D. 2006. *Healing psychiatry: Bridging the science/humanism divide*. Cambridge: MIT Press.

Breuer, J., and Freud, S. 1955. Studies in hysteria. In J. Strachey, ed., *The standard edition of the complete psychological works of Sigmund Freud*, 2:1–241. London: Hogarth Press.

Brody, H. 2003. *Stories of sickness*. Oxford: Oxford University Press.

Brooks, P. 1984. *Reading for the plot: Design and intention in narrative*. Cambridge: Harvard University Press.

Brown, L. 1994. *Subversive dialogues: Theory in feminist therapy*. New York: Basic Books.

Burke, K. 1954. *Permanence and change*. Berkeley: University of California Press.

Busch, F., Rudden, M., and Shapiro, T. 2004. *Psychodynamic treatment of depression*. Washington, DC: American Psychiatric Publishing.

Cameron. D. 2007. Biobabble. *Critical Inquiry* 49, no. 4: 124–29.

Campinha-Bacote, J. 1994. Cultural competence in psychiatric mental health nursing: A conceptual model. *Mental Health Nursing* 29, no. 1: 1–8.

Campo, R. 2005. The medical humanities: For lack of a better term. *Journal of the American Medical Association* 294, no. 9: 1009–11.

Caplan, P. 1995. *They say you are crazy: How the world's most powerful psychiatrists decide who's normal.* Reading, MA: Perseus Books.

Carroll, L. 1992. *Alice's adventures in wonderland and through the looking glass.* New York: Knopf.

Cassel, E. 1982. The nature of suffering and the goals of medicine. *New England Journal of Medicine* 306, no. 11: 639–45.

Cazeaux, C. 2007. *Metaphor and continental philosophy: From Kant to Derrida.* New York: Routledge.

Charmaz, K. 1991. *Good days, bad days: The self in chronic illness and time.* New Brunswick, NJ: Rutgers University Press.

Charon, R. 2001. Narrative medicine: A model for empathy, reflection, profession, and trust. *Journal of the American Medical Association* 286, no. 15: 1897–1902.

———. 2004. Narrative and medicine. *New England Journal of Medicine* 350, no. 9: 862–64.

———. 2005. Narrative medicine: Attention, representation, affiliation. *Narrative* 13, no. 3: 261–70.

———. 2006. *Narrative medicine: Honoring the stories of illness.* Oxford: Oxford University Press.

Chekhov, A. 1967. *Ivanov.* In *The Oxford Chekov,* vol. 2, translated and edited by R. Hingley, 163–228. London: Oxford University Press.

———. 1997. *Anton Chekhov's life and thought: Selected letters and commentaries.* Translated by M. H. Heim, in collaboration with S. Karlinsky. Selection, introduction, and commentary by S. Karlinsky. Evanston, IL: Northwestern University Press.

———. 2004. *A life in letters.* Edited by R. Bartlett, translated by R. Bartlett and A. Phillip. London: Penguin Books.

Coles, R. 1975. *The Mind's Fate: Ways of seeing psychiatry and psychoanalysis.* Boston: Little, Brown and Co.

———. 1995. *The mind's fate: A psychiatrist looks at his profession.* Boston: Little, Brown and Co.

———. 2002. Foreword. In J. Coulehan, ed., *Chekhov's doctors: A collection of Chekhov's medical tales,* ix–xii. Kent, OH: Kent State University Press.

Comas-Diaz, L. 1994. An integrative approach. In L. Comas-Diaz and B. Green, eds., *Women of color: Integrating ethnic and gender identities in psychotherapy,* 287–318. New York: Guilford Press.

————. 2000. An ethnopolitical approach to working with people of color. *American Psychologist* 55, November: 1319–1325.

Coope, J. 1997. *Doctor Chekhov: A study in literature and medicine.* Chale, Isle of Wight: Cross.

Corsini, R. 2005. Introduction. In R. Corsini and D. Wedding, eds., *Current psychotherapies,* 7th ed., 1–15. Southbank, Australia: Thomson.

Corsini, R., and Wedding, D., eds. 2005. *Current psychotherapies,* 7th ed. Southbank, Australia: Thomson.

Coulehan, J. 1997. "Ivanov." Literature, Arts, and Medicine Database. http://litmed.med.nyu.edu/Annotation?action=view&annid=1139 (accessed January 7, 2006).

————, ed. 2002. *Chekhov's doctors: A collection of Chekhov's medical tales.* Kent, OH: Kent State University Press.

Crossley, M. 2000. *Introducing narrative psychology: Self, trauma, and the construction of meaning.* Buckingham, UK: Open University Press.

Davis, L. 2007. *Obsession: A history.* Chicago: University of Chicago Press.

Davis, L., and Morris, D. 2007. Biocultures manifesto. *New Literary History* 38:411–18.

del Vecchio, P. 2006. All we are saying is give people with mental illness a chance. *Psychiatric Services* 57, no. 5: 646.

Dittrich, L., ed. 2003. The humanities and medicine: Reports of 41 U.S., Canadian, and international programs. *Academic Medicine* 78:951–1074.

Divakaruni, C. 1999. Mrs. Dutta writes a letter. In A. Tan, ed., *The Best American Short Stories, 1999,* 29–48. Boston: Houghton Mifflin.

Double, D. 2006. *Critical psychiatry: The limits of madness.* New York: Palgrave.

Du Gay, P., Evans, J., and Redman, P., eds. 2000. *Identity: A reader.* London: Sage Publications.

Duncan, B. 2002a. The founder of common factors: An interview with Saul Rosenzweig. *Journal of Psychotherapy Integration* 12, no. 1: 10–31.

————. 2002b. The legacy of Saul Rosenzweig: The profundity of the Dodo bird. *Journal of Psychotherapy Integration* 12, no. 1: 32–57.

Duncan, B., and Miller, S. 2000. The client's theory of change. *Journal of Psychotherapy Integration* 10, no. 1: 169–87.

Edwards, D. 2004. *Art therapy.* London: Sage Publications.

Engel, G. 1977. The need for a new medical model: A challenge for biomedicine. *Science* 196, no. 4286: 129–36.

————. 1980. The clinical application of the biopsychosocial model. *American Journal of Psychiatry* 137, no. 5: 535–44.

Enns, C. 2004. *Feminist theories and feminist psychotherapies.* New York: Haworth Press.

Everett, A. 2005. AACP well represented in SAMHSA recovery consensus conference. *Community Psychiatrist* 19, no. 1: 3.

Farber, S. 1993. *Madness, heresy, and the rumor of angels: The revolt against the mental health system*. Chicago: Open Court.

Finke, M. 2005. *Seeing Chekhov: Life and art*. Ithaca, NY: Cornell University Press.

Fishman, D., and Franks, C. 1992. Evolution and differentiation within behavioral therapy: A theoretical and epistemological review. In D. Freedheim, ed., *History of psychotherapy: A century of change*, 159–97. Washington, DC: American Psychological Association.

Flax, J. 1990. *Thinking fragments: Psychoanalysis, feminism, and postmodernism*. Berkeley: University of California Press.

Flexner, A. 1910. *Medical education in the United States and Canada: A report to the Carnegie Foundation for the Advancement of Science*. New York: Carnegie Foundation for the Advancement of Teaching.

Foucault, M. 1988a. The ethics of care for the self as a practice and freedom. In J. Bernauer and D. Rasmussen, ed., *The final Foucault*, 1–20. Cambridge: MIT Press.

———. 1988b. Technologies of the self. In L. Martin, H. Gutman, and P. Hutton, eds., *Technologies of the self: A seminar with Michel Foucault*, 16–49. Amherst: University of Massachusetts Press.

Frank, A. 1992. *At the will of the body: Reflections on illness*. Boston: Houghton Mifflin.

———. 1995. *The wounded storyteller: Body, illness, and ethics*. Chicago: University of Chicago Press.

Frank, J., and Frank, J. 1991. *Persuasion and healing: A comparative study of psychotherapy*. Baltimore: Johns Hopkins University Press.

Franzen, J. 2001. *The corrections*. New York: Farrar, Straus and Giroux.

Freedman, J., and Combs, G. 1996. *Narrative therapy: The social construction of preferred realities*. New York: W. W. Norton.

Freud, S. 1953. Interpretation of dreams. In J. Strachey, ed., *The standard edition of the complete psychological works of Sigmund Freud*, 20-21:1–629. London: Hogarth Press.

———. 1955. Studies on hysteria. In J. Strachey, ed., *The standard edition of the complete psychological works of Sigmund Freud*, 2:1–335. London: Hogarth Press.

———. 1958. Remembering, repeating and working-through. In J. Strachey, ed., *The standard edition of the complete psychological works of Sigmund Freud*, 12:147–56. London: Hogarth Press.

———. 1959. An autobiographical study. In J. Strachey, ed., *The standard edition of the complete psychological works of Sigmund Freud Sigmund Freud*, 20:3–71. London: Hogarth Press.

Friedland, L., ed. 1964. *Letters on the short story, the drama, and other literary topics, by Anton Chekhov.* New York: Benjamin Blom.

Fulford, K. W. M. 2004. Facts/values: Ten principles of values-based medicine. In J. Radden, ed., *The philosophy of psychiatry: A companion,* 205–236. Oxford: Oxford University Press.

Fulford, K. W. M., Morris, K., Sadler, J., and Stanghellini, G. 2003a. *Nature and narrative: An introduction to the new philosophy of psychiatry.* Oxford: Oxford University Press.

Fulford, K. W. M., Morris, K., Sadler, J., and Stanghellini, G. 2003b. Past improbable, future possible: The renaissance in philosophy and psychiatry. In K. W. M. Fulford, K. Morris, J. Sadler, and G. Stanghellini, eds. *Nature and narrative: An introduction to the new philosophy of psychiatry,* 1–41. Oxford: Oxford University Press.

Fulford, K. W. M., Thornton, T., and Graham, G. 2006. *Oxford textbook of philosophy and psychiatry.* Oxford: Oxford University Press.

Geertz, C. 1973. *The interpretation of cultures.* New York: Basic Books.

Ghaemi, S. N. 2003. *The concepts of psychiatry: A pluralistic approach to the mind and mental illness.* Baltimore: Johns Hopkins University Press.

Giddens, A. 1991. *Modernity and self-identity: Self and society in contemporary life.* New York: Basic Books.

Gilman, R. 1995. *Chekhov's plays: An opening to eternity.* New Haven: Yale University Press.

Goffman, E. 1961. *Asylums: Essays on the social situation of mental patients and other inmates.* New York: Doubleday.

Gold, J., and Stricker, G. 2006. Introduction: An overview of psychotherapy integration. In G. Stricker and J. Gold, eds., *A casebook of psychotherapy integration,* 3–16. Washington, DC: American Psychological Association.

Goldenberg, I., and Goldenberg, H. 2005. Family therapy. In R. Corsini and D. Wedding, eds., *Current psychotherapies,* 7th ed., 372–405. Belmont, CA: Brooks/Cole–Thomson.

Greenberg, G. 2010. *Manufacturing Depression: The History of a Modern Disease.* New York: Simon and Schuster.

Greenberg, R. 1999. Common psychosocial factors in psychiatric drug therapy. In M. Hubble, B. Duncan, and S. Miller, eds., *The heart and soul of change: What works in therapy,* 297–328. Washington, DC: American Psychological Association.

Greenhalgh, T. 1999. Narrative based medicine in an evidenced based world. *British Medical Journal* 318:323–25.

Gurman, A., and Lebow, G. 2005. Family therapy and couple therapy. In B. Sadock and V. Sadock, eds., *Kaplan and Sadock's comprehensive text-*

book of psychiatry, 8th ed., 2584–96. Philadelphia: Lippincott Williams andWilkins.

Gurman, A., and Messer, S., eds. 2003. *Essential psychotherapies: Theory and practice*, 2d ed. New York: Guilford Press.

Guzder, J., and Krishna, M. 2005. Mind the gap: Diaspora issues of Indian origin women in psychotherapy. *Psychology and developing societies* 17, no. 2: 121–138.

Hall, S. 1996. Introduction: Who needs identity. In S. Hall and P. du Gay, eds., *Questions of cultural identity*, 1–17. London: Sage Publications.

Hall, S., and du Gay, P., eds. 1996. *Questions of cultural identity*. London: Sage Publications.

Hanisch, C. 1971. The personal is political. In J. Agel, ed., *Radical therapist: The radical therapist collection*, 152–157. New York: Ballantine Books.

Hare, D. 1997. Introduction to *Ivanov: A play in four acts*. Adapted by D. Hare, vii–xi. London: Methuen Drama.

Hawkins, A. H. 1993. *Reconstructing illness: Studies in pathography*. West Lafayette, IN: Purdue University Press.

Hawkins, A. H., and McEntyre, M. C., eds. 2000. *Teaching literature and medicine*. New York: Modern Language Association.

Hesse, M. 2000. The explanatory function of metaphor. In J. McErlean, ed., *Philosophies of science: From foundations to contemporary issues*, 349–55. Belmont, California: Wadsworth.

Hiatt, M. 1999. Around the continent in 180 days: The controversial journey of Abraham Flexner. *Pharos* 62, Winter: 18–24.

Hingley, R. 1976. *A new life of Anton Chekhov*. New York: Knopf.

Hogan, M. F. 2003. The President's New Freedom Commission: Recommendations to transform mental health care in America. *Psychiatric Services* 54, no. 11: 1467–74.

Holt, T. 2004. Narrative medicine and negative capability. *Literature and Medicine* 23, no. 2: 318–33.

Hopper, K. 2007. Rethinking social recovery in schizophrenia: What a capabilities approach might offer. *Social Science and Medicine* 65, no. 5: 868–79.

Hoshmand, L. 2000. Narrative psychology. In E. Kazdin, ed., *Encyclopedia of psychology*, 382–87. Washington, DC: American Psychological Association.

Hubble, M., Duncan, B., and Miller, S., eds. 1999. *The heart and soul of change: What works in therapy*. Washington, DC: American Psychological Association.

Huber, C. 1999. *The depression book: Depression as an opportunity for spiritual growth*. Murphys, CA: Keep It Simple Books.

Humm, M., ed. 1992. *Modern feminisms: Political, literary, cultural*. New York: Columbia University Press.

Hunter, K. M. 1991. *Doctors' stories: The narrative structure of medical knowledge*. Princeton: Princeton University Press.

Husserl, E. 1970. Philosophy and the crisis of European humanity. In J. Wild, ed., *The crisis of European sciences and transcendental phenomenology*, 269–301. Evanston, IL: Northwestern University Press.

Huxley, A. 1945. *The perennial philosophy*. New York: Harper and Brothers.

Jack, D. C. 1991. *Silencing the self: Women and depression*. Cambridge: Harvard University Press.

James, W. 1982. *The varieties of religious experience*. Harmondsworth: Penguin Classics.

Jaspers, K. 1981. Philosophical autobiography. In P. Schilpp, ed., *The philosophy of Karl Jaspers*. La Salle, IL: Open Court.

———. 1997. *General psychopathology*. Translated by J. Hoenig and M. Hamilton. Baltimore: Johns Hopkins University Press.

Jayakar, K. 1994. Women of the Indian subcontinent. In L. Comas-Diaz and B. Green, eds., *Women of color: Integrating ethnic and gender identities in psychotherapy*, 161–182. New York: Guilford Press.

Jensen, J. P., Bergin, A. E., and Greaves, D. W. 1990. The meaning of eclecticism: New survey and analysis of components. *Professional Psychology: Research and Practice* 21:124–30.

Jones, A. H., ed. 1991. *Literature and medicine: Tenth anniversary retrospective*. Baltimore: Johns Hopkins University Press.

Kandel, E. 1998. A new intellectual framework for psychiatry. *American Journal of Psychiatry* 155, no. 5: 457–69.

Kataev, V. 2002. *If only we could know! An interpretation of Chekhov*. Translated and edited by H. Pitcher. Chicago: Ivan R. Dee.

Kessler, R. C., Berglund, P., Demler, O., Jin, R., Koretz, D., Merikangas, K. R., Rush, J., Walters, E. E., and Wang, P. S. 2003. The epidemiology of major depressive disorder: Results from the national comorbidity survey replication. *Journal of the American Medical Association* 289, no. 23: 3095–3105.

Khanna, R. 1996. The write spirit. *Life Positive*, September www.lifepositive.com/mind/personal-growth/write-therapy/write.asp (accessed October 9, 2008).

Kirklin, D., and Richardson, R., eds. 2001. *Medical humanities: A practical introduction*. London: Royal College of Physicians.

Kirsch, I., Moore, T., Scoboria, A., and Nicholls, S. 2002. The emperor's new drugs: An analysis of antidepressant medication data submitted to the U.S. Food and Drug Administration. *Prevention and Treatment* 5. www.journals.apa.org/prevention/volume5/toc-jul15-02.html (accessed June 2, 2005).

Klein, D., and Wender, P. 2005. *Understanding depression: A complete guide to its diagnosis and treatment,* 2nd ed. Oxford: Oxford University Press.

Kleinman, A. 1988. *The illness narratives: Suffering, healing and the human condition*. New York: Basic Books.

Klerman, G., Weissman, M., Rounsaville, B., and Chevron, E. 1984. *Interpersonal psychotherapy of depression*. New York: Basic Books.

Kramer, K. 1979. Stories of ambiguity. In R. Matlaw, ed., *Anton Chekhov's short stories: Texts of the stories, backgrounds, and criticism*, 338–51. New York: W. W. Norton.

Kramer, P. 1997. What Ivanov needs in the 90's is an anti-depressant. *New York Times*, December 21, sec. 2.

———. 2005. *Against depression*. New York: Viking.

Kristeva, J. 1989. *Black sun: Depression and melancholia*. New York: Columbia University Press.

Lacasse, J. R., and Leo, J. 2005. Serotonin and depression: A disconnect between the advertisements and the scientific literature. *PLoS Medicine* 2, no. 12: 1–6.

Laing, R. D. 1967. *The politics of experience*. New York: Pantheon Books.

———. 1968. The obvious. In D. Cooper, ed., *The dialectics of liberation*, 13–34. Harmondsworth: Penguin.

Lakoff, G., and Johnson, M. 1980. *Metaphors we live by*. Chicago: University of Chicago Press.

Lambert, M. J. 1992. Implications of outcome research for psychotherapy integration. In J. C. Norcross and M. R. Goldfried, eds., *Handbook of psychotherapy integration*, 94–129. New York: Basic Books.

———. 2007. Presidential address: What we have learned from a decade of research aimed at improving psychotherapy outcome in routine care. *Psychotherapy Research* 17, no. 1: 1–14.

Lambert, M. J., and Bergin, A. 1994. The effectiveness of psychotherapy. In A. E. Bergin and S. L. Garfield, eds., *Handbook of psychotherapy and behavior change*, 143–49. New York: Wiley.

Lane, C. 2007. *Shyness: How normal behavior became a sickness*. New Haven: Yale University Press.

Law, J., and Mol, A., eds. 2002. *Complexities: Social studies of knowledge practices*. Durham, NC: Duke University Press.

Lewis, B. 2006a. A mad fight: Psychiatry and disability activism. In L. Davis, ed., *Disability studies reader*, 2d ed., 339–366. New York: Routledge.

———. 2006b. *Moving beyond Prozac, DSM, and the new psychiatry: The birth of postpsychiatry*. Ann Arbor: University of Michigan Press.

———. 2007. The biopsychosocial model and philosophic pragmatism: Is George Engel a pragmatist? *Philosophy, Psychiatry, and Psychology* 14, no. 4: 299–310.

———. 2009. Madness studies. *Literature and Medicine* 28, no. 1: 152–171.

Luborsky, L., Rosenthal, R., Diguer, L., Andrusyna, T., Berman, J. S., Levitt, J. T., Seligman, D., and Krause, E. 2002. The dodo bird verdict is alive and well=mmostly. *Clinical Psychology: Science and Practice* 9, no. 1: 2–12.

Luborsky, L., Singer, B., and Luborsky, L. 1975. Comparative studies of psychotherapies: Is it true that "everyone has won and all must have prizes"? *Archives of General Psychiatry* 32:995–1008.

Luhrmann, T. M. 2000. *Of two minds: An anthropologists looks at American psychiatry.* New York: Vintage Books.

MacFarquhar, L. 2007. Two heads: A marriage devoted to the mind-body problem. *New Yorker*, February 12: 82, 49, 58–69.

Mansfield, N. 2000. *Subjectivity: Theories of the self from Freud to Haraway.* New York: New York University Press.

Martin, E. 2006. The pharmaceutical person. *BioSocieties* 1:273–87.

———. 2007. *Biopolar expeditions: Mania and depression in American culture.* Princeton: Princeton University Press.

Martin, P. 1999. *The Zen path through depression.* San Francisco: HarperSanFancisco.

Martin, W. 1986. *Recent theories of narrative.* Ithaca, NY: Cornell University Press.

Martinez, R. 2002. Narrative understanding and methods in psychiatry and behavioral health. In R. Charon and M. Montello, eds., *Stories matter: The role of narrative in medical ethics*, 126–37. New York: Routledge.

Mayberg, H. 2004. Depression: A neuropsychiatric perspective. In J. Panskepp, ed., *Textbook of biological psychiatry*, 197–229. Wilmington, DE: Wiley-Liss.

McHugh, P. R. 1992. A structure for psychiatry at the century's turn: The view from Johns Hopkins. *Journal of the Royal Society of Medicine* 85:483–87.

McHugh, P. R., and P. R. Slavney. 1998. *The perspectives of psychiatry,* 2d ed. Baltimore: Johns Hopkins University Press.

McWhinney, I. 1986. Are we on the brink of a major transformation in clinical method? *Canadian Medical Association Journal* 135:873–78.

Messud, C. 2006. *The emperor's children.* New York: Vintage Books.

Meyer, A. 1957. *Psychobiology: A science of man.* Springfield, IL: Charles C. Thomas.

Moncrieff, J., and Kirsch, I. 2005. Efficacy of antidepressants in adults. *British Medical Journal* 331:155–57.

Morrison, L. 2005. *Talking back to psychiatry: The consumer/survivor/ex-patient movement.* New York: Routledge.

Nadeson, M. 2005. *Constructing autism: Unraveling the "truth" and understanding the social.* New York: Routlege.

Norcross, J. C., and Beutler, L. E. 2008. Integrative psychotherapies. In R. Corsini and D. Wedding, eds., *Current psychotherapies*, 8th ed., 481–511. Belmont, CA: Brooks/Cole–Thomson.

Norcross, J. C., Karpiak, C. P., and Santoro, S. O. 2005. Clinical psychologists across the years: The division of clinical psychology, 1960–2003. *Journal of Clinical Psychology* 61:1587–94.

Norman, R. A. 2005. Literature and medicine. *Dermanities* 3, no. 2. www .dermanities.com/detail.asp?article=171 (accessed January 2, 2006).

Odegaard, C. 1986. *Dear doctor: A personal letter to a physician.* Menlo Park, CA: Henry Kaiser Foundation.

Ogles, B., Anderson, T., and Lunnen, K. 1999. The contributions of models and techniques to therapeutic efficacy. In M. Hubble, B. Duncan, and S. Miller, eds., *The heart and soul of change: What works in therapy,* 201–225. Washington, DC: American Psychological Association.

Orr, J. 2006. *Panic diaries: A genealogy of panic disorders.* Durham, NC: Duke University Press.

Pellegrino, E. 1979. *Humanism and the physician.* Knoxville: University of Tennessee Press.

———. 1982. Being ill and being healed: Some reflections on the grounding of medical morality. In V. Kestenbaum, ed., *The humanity of the ill: Phenomenological perspectives,* 157–66. Knoxville: University of Tennessee Press.

Phillips, J. 1999. The psychodynamic narrative. In G. Roberts and J. Holmes, eds., *Healing stories: Narrative in psychiatry and psychotherapy,* 27–48. Oxford: Oxford University Press.

———. 2004. Understanding/explanation. In J. Radden, ed., *The philosophy of psychiatry: A companion,* 180–191. Oxford: Oxford University Press.

Pierce, C. M., and Allen, G. B. 1975. Childism. *Psychiatric Annals* 5:266–70.

Pollock, G. 1978. Process and affect: Mourning and grief. *International Journal of Psychoanalysis* 59:255–76.

———. 1989. *The mourning-liberation process.* Madison, CT: International Universities Press.

Popkin, C. 1993. *The pragmatics of insignificance: Chekhov, Zoshchenko, Gogol.* Stanford: Stanford University Press.

Porter, R. 2002. *Madness: A brief history.* Oxford: Oxford University Press.

Puustinen, R. 1999. Baktin's philosophy and medical practice: Toward a semiotic theory of doctor-patient interaction. *Medicine, Health Care and Philosophy* 2:275–81.

———. 2000. Voices to be heard: The many positions of a physician in Anton Chekhov's short story. A case history. *Journal of Medical Ethics* 26:37–42.

Quitkin, F. M., Rabkin, J., Gerald, J., Davis, J., and Klein, D. 2000. Validity of clinical trials of antidepressants. *American Journal of Psychiatry* 157:327–37.

Radden, J., ed. 2004. *The philosophy of psychiatry: A companion.* Oxford: Oxford University Press.

Rampton, S., and Stauber, J. 2002. *Trust us we're experts: How industry manipulates science and gambles with your future*. New York: Tarcher.

Raskin, N., and Rogers, C. 2005. Person-centered therapy. In R. Corsini and D. Wedding, eds., *Current psychotherapies*, 7th ed., 238–69. Belmont, CA: Brooks/Cole–Thomson.

Rayfield, D. 1997. *Anton Chekhov: A life*. London: HarperCollins.

Rice, L., and Greenberg, L. 1992. Humanistic approaches to psychology. In D. Freedheim, ed., *History of psychotherapy: A century of change*, 197–225. Washington, DC: American Psychological Association.

Richert, A. 2006. Narrative psychology and psychotherapy integration. *Journal of Psychotherapy Integration* 16, no. 1: 84–110.

Ricoeur, P. 1977. *The rule of metaphor: Multi-disciplinary studies in the creation of meaning in language*. Toronto: University of Toronto Press.

———. 1984. *Time and narrative*. Vol 1. Chicago: University of Chicago Press.

———. 1991a. *From text to action: Essays in hermeneutics, II*. Evanston, IL: Northwestern University Press.

———. 1991b. Life in quest of narrative. In D. Wood, ed., *On Paul Ricoeur: Narrative and interpretation*, 20–33. London: Routledge.

———. 1991c. Word, polysemy, metaphor: Creativity in language. In M. Valdes, ed., *A Ricoeur reader: Reflection and imagination*, 65–85. Toronto: University of Toronto Press.

———. 1992. *Oneself as another*. Chicago: University of Chicago Press.

Roberts, G., and Holmes, J. 1999. *Healing stories: Narrative psychiatry and psychotherapy*. Oxford: Oxford University Press.

Rogers, C. 1961. *On becoming a person*. Boston: Houghton Mifflin.

Rose, N. 2003. Neurochemical selves. *Society* 41, November–December: 46–59.

Rosenzweig, S. 1936. Some implicit common factors in diverse methods of psychotherapy: At last the Dodo said, "Everybody has won and all must have prizes." *American Journal of Orthopsychiatry* 6:412–15.

Rutherford, B., and Hellerstein, D. 2008. Divergent fates of the medical humanities in psychiatry and internal medicine: Should psychiatry be rehumanized? *Academic Medicine* 32:206–13.

Rubovits-Seitz, P. 1998. *Depth-psychological understanding: The methodologic grounding of clinical interpretation*. Hillsdale, NJ: Analytic Press.

Sadler, J. 2004. *Values and psychiatric disorders*. Oxford: Oxford University Press.

SAMHSA. 2006. *National consensus statement on mental health recovery*. Rockville, MD. Available at www.mentalhealth.samhsa.gov/publications/allpubs/sma05-4129 (accessed July 7, 2010).

Scheff, T. 1999. *Being mentally ill: A sociological theory*. Chicago: Aldine Press.

Schreurs, A. 2002. *Psychotherapy and spirituality: Integrating the spiritual dimension into therapeutic practice*. London: Jessica Kingsley Publishers.

See, C. 2002. *Making a literary life: Advice for writers and other dreamers*. New York: Ballantine Books.

Shaffer, J. 1978. *Humanistic psychology*. Upper Saddle River, NJ: Prentice Hall.

Shorter, E. 1997. *A History of psychiatry: From the era of the asylum to the age of Prozac*. New York: John Wiley and Sons.

Smith, R. 2005. Medical journals are an extension of the marketing arm of pharmaceutical companies. *PLoS Medicine* 2, no. 5: 364–66.

Softky, E. 1997. Cross-cultural understanding spiced with the Indian diaspora. *Black Issues in Higher Education* 14, no. 15: 26–27.

Solomon, A. 2001. *The noonday demon: An atlas of depression*. New York: Scribner.

Sontag, S. 1978. *Illness as metaphor*. New York: Farrar, Straus and Giroux.

Sowers, W. 2005. Recovery and equity: The time is now. *Community Psychiatrist* 19, no. 1: 1–2.

Sowers, W., and Thompson, K., eds. 2007. *Keystones for collaboration and leadership: Issues and recommendations for the transformation of community psychiatry*. Available at www.communitypsychiatry.org/aacp/Transformationof PsychiatryReport.pdf. July 7, 2010.

Spitzer, R., Skodol, A., Gibbon, M., and Williams, J. 1981. *DSM-III casebook*. Washington, DC: American Psychiatric Association.

Strawson, G. 2004. Against narrativity. *Ratio* 18, December 4: 429–52.

Szasz, T. 1974. *The myth of mental illness: Foundations of a theory personal conduct*. New York: Harper and Row.

Tallman, K., and Bohart, A. 1999. The client as a common factor: Clients as self-healers. In M. Hubble, B. Duncan, and S. Miller, eds., *The heart and soul of change: What works in therapy*, 91–133. Washington, DC: American Psychological Association.

Tamini, S., and Cohen, C., eds. 2008. *Liberatory psychiatry*. Cambridge: Cambridge University Press.

Taylor, C. 2002. *Varieties of religion today*. Cambridge: Harvard University Press.

Thompson, K. 2006. Keynote address. American Association of Community Psychiatrists, Winter Meeting, Pittsburgh, PA.

Toombs, K. 2001. Introduction: Phenomenology and medicine. In K. Toombs, ed., *Handbook of phenomenology and medicine*, 1–26. Dordrecht, Netherlands: Kluwer Academic Publishers.

Tucker, W. M. 1994. Teaching psychiatry through literature: The short story as case history. *Academic Psychiatry* 18:211–19.

Tyrer, P., and Steinberg, P. 2005. *Models for mental disorder*, 4th ed. Chichester, England: John Wiley and Sons.

Valle, R. 1989. The emergence of transpersonal psychology. In R. Valle and S. Halling, eds., *Existential-phenomenological perspectives on psychology*, 257–268. New York: Plenum Press.

Valenstein, E. 1998. *Blaming the brain: The truth about drugs and mental health*. New York: Free Press.

Verghese, A. 2001. The physician as storyteller. *Annals of Internal Medicine* 135, no. 11: 1012–17.

Wallace, E. 1994. Psychiatry and its nosology: A historico-philosophical overview. In J. Sadler, O. Wiggins, and M. Schwartz, eds., *Philosophical perspectives on psychiatric diagnostic classification*, 16–89. Baltimore: Johns Hopkins University Press.

Wampold, B. E. 2001. *The great psychotherapy debate*. Mahwah, NJ: Lawrence Erlbaum Associates.

———. 2006. Not a scintilla of evidence to support empirically supported treatments as more effective than other treatments. In J. C. Norcross, L. E. Beutler, and R. F. Levant, eds., *Evidence-based practices in mental health: Debate and dialogue on the fundamental questions*, 299–307. Washington, DC: American Psychological Association.

Watson, J. B. 1913. Psychology as the behaviorist views it. *Psychological Review* 10:158–77.

Weintraub, A. 2004. *Yoga for depression*. New York: Broadway Books.

White, M. 2007. *Maps of narrative practice*. New York: W. W. Norton.

White, M., and Epston, D. 1990. *Narrative means to therapeutic ends*. New York: W. W. Norton.

Wilfley, D. 2005. Interpersonal psychotherapy. In B. Sadock and V. Sadock, eds., *Kaplan and Sadock's comprehensive textbook of psychiatry*, 8th ed., 2611–20. Philadelphia: Lippincott Williams and Wilkins.

Wood, M. 2004. "I found him!": Diagnostic narrative in *The DSM-IV Casebook*. *Narrative* 12, no 2: 195–220.

World Health Organization. Depression. www.who.int/mental_health/management/depression/definition/en (accessed May 27, 2006).

Zaner, R. 1990. Medicine and dialogue. *Journal of Medicine and Philosophy* 15:303–25.

Zaretsky, E. 2005. *Secrets of the soul: A social and cultural history of psychoanalysis*. New York: Vintage Books.

Andreasen, Nancy, 57, 61, 89
Angell, Marcia, 62–63
Antipsychiatry, ix, 62, 64, 137, 151

Bakhtin, Michael, 6
Barthes, Roland, 47, 192
Beck, Aron, 94–97
Biobabble, 169
Biocultures, 189n2
Bioethics, xvi, 31, 152, 156, 170
Biopsychiatry: dogmatism and, 11,
    193n3; model of treatment, 88–98,
    102; moving beyond, 171–72; phar-
    maceutical industry and, 61–64;
    reductionism and, 1–3, 15–16,
    168–69; shift from psychoanalysis,
    ix–xi, 193n1
Biopsychosocial model, 8, 20, 31,
    161–62, 193n1, 194n4
Bordo, Susan, 8
Braken, Pat, ix, 153, 155–56
Brody, Howard, 26
Brooks, Peter, 47–58
Brown, Laura, 142–43

Carrol, Lewis, 40
Case examples, 78
Cassel, Eric, 29
Character, 13, 43, 47–49, 52, 69, 160
Charmaz, Kathy, 25
Charon, Rita, 28–30

Chekhov, Anton, xiii, 1–17, 65, 151,
    157
Chemical imbalance, 5, 61, 89–91,
    148, 165, 189n1
Childism, 51–52
Coles, Robert, 65–66, 189n3, 193nn1, 3
Comos-Diaz, Lillian, 139–40
Consumer movement, 63, 153
Corrections, The (Franzen), 71
Creativity, 129–35, 154, 156
Cultural competence, 136–37

Dark night of the soul, 126–27
Davis, Lennard, xi, 189n2
del Vecchio, Paulo, 155
Diagnostic and Statistical Manual of
    Mental Disorders (DSM-III), ix, 61,
    75–77
Disability, 153
Discourse, xii, 2, 15, 64
Disease/illness distinction, 67–70,
    73–74
Divakaruni, Chitra, xv, 82–83, 86, 90,
    134–35, 144, 157, 173
Dodo bird verdict, 37–42, 52, 55, 159

Eclecticism, 41–42, 52, 163
Edson, Margaret, 30–31
Emperor's Children (Messud) 48–50, 80
Engel, George, 20, 29, 193n1
Evidence-based practice, 52, 147, 158

Feminism, 138
Flexner, Abraham, 19–25, 28, 30
Frank, Arthur, 25–26, 54
Frank, Jerome, 38–39
Franzen, Jonathan, 71
Freud, Sigmund, 14, 33, 58–61,
    99–100, 130
Fulford, K. W., 147, 171
Future histories, 80–82

Geertz, Clifford, 76
Gender, 137–42
Ghaemi, Nassir, ix, 190n13, 192n19,
    193n1
Giddens, Anthony, 53
Goffman, Erving, 137
Goldenberg, Irene and Herbert,
    109–12
Greenberg, Gary, xii

Hall, Stuart, 48
Hanish, Carol, 137–38
Hawkins, Anne Hunsaker, 27–28
Health care crisis, 22
Hesse, Mary, 43–44, 70, 87
Hopper, Kim, 153
Huber, Chris, 125–26
Humanistic psychology, 35, 121
Hunter, Kathryn Montgomery, 13, 27
Husserl, Edmund, 21–22, 60

Ivanov (Chekhov), xiii, xv, 1–18, 157

Jack, Dana Crowley, 138–39
James, William, 126–28
Jaspers, Karl, 59–63, 68, 171–72

Kandel, Eric, 88
Klein, Donald, 89–92, 159

Kleinman, Arthur, 24–25
Klerman, Gerald, 104–6
Kramer, Peter, 5–6, 14

Laing, R. D., 137
Lakoff, George, 43
Lambert, Michael, 37, 54
Lane, Christopher, xi–xii
Life politics, 53, 56
Literary case histories, xv, 78–79
Literature and medicine, 3, 20, 26–28
Luhrmann, T. M., ix–x, 77, 87

Martin, Emily, xiii, 71–72
Martin, Philip, 123–25
McHugh, Paul, vii, 193n1
McWhinney, Ian, 20
Medical anthropology, 24
Medical sociology, 24
Medication, vii, 56, 68–73, 84, 92–93,
    145–48, 163
Medicine, history of, 18–28
Meditation, 122–27, 131, 164
Messud, Claire, 48–50, 80
Metaphor, 43–45, 70, 75, 85, 165
Models of mental illness, 81,
    87–88
Mrs. Dutta Writes a Letter (Divaka-
    runi), 82–150, 157, 159, 162–93

Narrative: medicine, xiv, 18–31, 57,
    64–74, 83, 145, 152, 156; multi-
    plicity, 14–16, 191n18; psychiatry,
    57–75, 144–73; psychotherapy, xiv,
    32–56, 64–68, 83, 194n4
Narrative identity, 43, 82, 86, 165;
    character and, 47–59; disease/illness
    and, 70; models of mental illness
    and, 92, 120, 143, 145, 148–49;

psychoanalysis and, 33; Ricoeur and, xiii, 88

Narrative theory, vii, xii–xiv, 158; case examples and, 75, 81–82, 86, 103; disease/illness and, 68; psychotherapy and, 32, 36, 42–55; psychotherapy integration and, 151

Neuroscience, 18, 71–72, 168–69

Nido therapy, 136

Orr, Jackie, xii

Paradigm, ix–xii, 24, 62, 154–55, 168

Pelligrino, Edmund, 21–25

Person-centered medicine, 20

Pharmaceutical industry, xi, 62–63, 160

Phenomenology, xiii, 21–23, 29, 31, 60, 115, 150

Plot, 13, 43, 166; literary case and, 80–82; narrative identity and, 48–49, 52, 102–3, 145, 148; narrative theory and, 45–46, 68–69

Point of view, 6, 12, 43, 49, 52, 75, 85, 160

Politics, 138

Pollock, George, 7, 99–102, 105

Postcolonial, 141–42

Postmodern, ix–xiii, 36, 39–41, 52, 165

Postpsychiatry, ix–xii, 63

Poststructuralism, xiii, 192nn18, 19

Power, xi–xii, 8, 39, 72, 139, 153

Prozac, 1

Psychiatry: history of, 57–64; philosophy and, xiii, 63, 171

Psychoanalysis, 171–72; dogmatism and, 193n3; history of, 32–35, 58–62; model of treatment, 98–103;

postmodern theory and, 39; shift from biopsychiatry, ix–xii, 193n1

Psychobabble, 169

Psychotherapy: cognitive-behavioral, 35, 93–98, 116, 121, 138, 144, 148, 156, 171; cultural, political, and feminist, 135–43; diversity, 36, 39–42, 52–53, 67; expressive, 129–35, 147, family, 36, 107–14, 145; history of, 33–42; humanistic, 35–36, 41, 53, 114–19, 121, 145, 148; integration, 32–33, 41–42, 52–57, 66–68, 74, 194; interpersonal, 104–7, 119, 135; research, 37–38; spiritual, 121–29, 145, 162

Race, 137, 141

Recovery movement, xvi, 64, 152–56

Reductionism, 2, 154, 168

Ricoeur, Paul, xii, 43–47, 81, 88, 158, 161, 163, 165

Rogers, Carl, 36, 114–19

Rose, Nicholas, 71–72

Sadler, John, ix

Selective serotonin reuptake inhibitors (SSRIs), 1

Sexism, 76, 140

Sontag, Susan, 70

Spiritual exile, 127–29

Szasz, Thomas, 137

Taylor, Charles, 127

Thomas, Phil, ix, 153

Thompson, Kenneth, 155

Toombs, Kay, 22

Transpersonal psychology, 121–27

Truth: biopsychiatry and, x; fiction and, 157; metaphor and, 44, 70;

Truth (*continued*)
  one vs. multiple, xv, 11–13, 144,
  170; relativism and, 151; values
  and, 39, 82, 154, 160

Valle, Ronald, 122
Values-based medicine, 147, 159
Verghese, Abraham, 12–13, 43, 65

Watson, J. B., 34
White, Michael, 50
Wit (Edson), 30–31

Yoga, 122–23, 126–27, 156

Zaner, Richard, 23
Zen Buddhism, 123–25

About the Author

Bradley Lewis, M.D., Ph.D., is associate professor at New York University's Gallatin School of Individualized Study with affiliated appointments in the Department of Psychiatry, the Department of Social and Cultural Analysis, and the Center for Bioethics. He has dual training in humanities and psychiatry, and he writes and teaches at the interface of medicine, humanities, and cultural studies. He is the author of *Moving beyond Prozac, DSM, and the New Psychiatry: The Birth of Postpsychiatry* and an associate editor for the *Journal of Medical Humanities*.